Dare
to dream

♥

My struggle to become a mum
– a story of heartache and hope

Dare to dream

IZZY JUDD

BANTAM PRESS

LONDON · TORONTO · SYDNEY · AUCKLAND · JOHANNESBURG

TRANSWORLD PUBLISHERS
61–63 Uxbridge Road, London W5 5SA
www.penguin.co.uk

Transworld is part of the Penguin Random House group of companies
whose addresses can be found at global.penguinrandomhouse.com

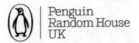
Penguin
Random House
UK

First published in Great Britain in 2017 by Bantam Press
an imprint of Transworld Publishers

A CIP catalogue record for this book
is available from the British Library.

ISBN 9780593078822

Typeset in Bembo/12pt by www.envyltd.co.uk
Printed and bound in Great Britain by Clays Ltd, St Ives plc

Penguin Random House is committed to a sustainable
future for our business, our readers and our planet. This book
is made from Forest Stewardship Council® certified paper.

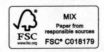
MIX
Paper from
responsible sources
FSC® C018179

1 3 5 7 9 10 8 6 4 2

For Harry & Lola ...
and all the stars that shine brighter.

Contents

Introduction

A problem shared

WHEN I WAS twenty-eight years old, I got married – a fairytale wedding to the man of my dreams. At the time of our wedding Harry and I had loved each other for many years, so we were fully ready to set up our lives together. The next step, for both of us, was to start a family. But that's not how our story went. I quickly found that, although I was young and healthy, I struggled to fall pregnant naturally.

There were some medical reasons given as to why I was having difficulties conceiving. I have Polycystic Ovarian Syndrome (PCOS) and was told that this was why I wasn't ovulating – but it didn't tell the whole story. I've always believed that my long struggle with anxiety, beginning when I was around thirteen years old, had a lot to do with it. The ways in which the mind and body work together are mysterious and powerful – they shape and influence each other. This of course can be both a good and a bad thing, as I was to discover.

Once I found out that conceiving naturally wasn't going to be straightforward, what followed were some very hard and lonely years. Even though they ended well with the birth of our beautiful daughter, Lola, in 2016, I'll never forget what we went through to have her.

During the years of waiting, I experienced so many emotions – from fear to frustration, desperation to anger, guilt to loneliness. Overall, I felt an overwhelming sadness and sense of responsibility that not only was I unable to give Harry the one thing we both wanted, I was also unable to give our parents grandchildren. My world stopped – it felt as if someone had pressed 'pause' and I couldn't move.

Of course, this story – or variations on it – is one that will be familiar to so many women. And yet through my own struggles there was hardly anything I read that gave me any comfort. Information on the science behind fertility treatment was easy to come by but I couldn't find anything that spoke to me on an emotional level, or that made sense of the complicated way I felt about myself, my body and what was happening to me.

After I'd had Lola, Harry and I had no problem in speaking openly about what we'd been through to conceive. In fact, we felt almost as if we had a duty to do so – we're in the public eye and we had the opportunity to draw attention to the fact that we'd had IVF with a wonderful result. I was amazed at the number of women who got in touch to let me know that hearing our story made a difference to them, that it had helped to hear that someone else had experienced what they were going through.

This led to my decision to write a book. I want to share my experiences and some of what I've learned, in the hope that it will help other women, and the friends and family who are supporting them during their fertility struggles. My greatest wish is that by telling my own story I can be a companion to others and help them to feel less alone – we're in this together.

I've included things that happened long before I ever thought about having a baby because I believe they had much to do with my struggle to conceive. As the philosopher Kierkegaard once said, 'Life can only be understood backwards; but it must be lived forwards.' I've lived my life forwards, of course, but it's only by looking back that I can fully understand some of what I've been through.

Not being able to fall pregnant isn't unusual or shameful – it's something that happens to so many of us. We'll all have our difficult moments in life, but when you feel you can't share them with others, they become even harder to deal with, as well as isolating. I hope that my words might give comfort to other women, and maybe start a more open conversation. Fertility is a very personal subject, one that needs to be approached with great sensitivity, but that doesn't mean that we just shouldn't talk about it.

Going through IVF is a lonely time. Even if you have a wonderful partner, as I do, and the support of family and close friends as, again, I did, it's still something very personal. It's *your* body that's injected, *your* hormones that are messed with, *your* cycle that's disrupted; *your* feelings of hope, disappointment, frustration and sorrow. And *your* challenge to bear that cycle of counting days, where a month can feel so long.

Everybody is unique and each woman will have her own individual set of issues and complications – the sliding scale of infertility is vast and covers a multitude of different things. I don't know exactly what other women go through, of course, but I know about the feelings that accompany so much of the struggle: the sense of isolation and failure; trying to manage the side effects from the drugs you have to take and the fear that you will never succeed in having a baby.

When I began to write, a part of me wondered whether my story was full enough. Did enough happen to me? Did I go through enough on my journey for a baby? I know there are women who undergo many more cycles of IVF than I did. But looking back at the many notes and diaries that I kept during the process, I realized just how much *did* happen to me, even in that fairly short space of time: the medication I took, the doctors I saw, the different things I tried. I remembered all over again how very real and very painful it was, and how slowly time seemed to pass.

There are things in this book that were tough to revisit in my mind and to write about, but they're important in telling the full story. Putting all the pieces of the puzzle together and looking back on it has been fascinating and therapeutic. I hope now that it will be useful to other women, however it compares to their journey.

This is my side of the story but it doesn't mean that Harry

wasn't with me every step of the way. Going through fertility treatment is all about teamwork. This is why Harry has written his side of the story for this book, too. He's always been completely involved, an equal partner in everything that we faced and very willing to talk about it. More than that, he's been a constant source of warmth, comfort and calm, always on my side. I felt he never cared about anything else other than me – it wasn't the outcome that mattered most, it was me.

If you're reading this and about to start fertility treatment, don't be frightened. IVF is amazing and magical. Take time to do the things that make you happy, deal with things one day at a time, and never give up hope. Look after yourself mentally and physically. Enjoy long walks and discover your own space where you can find peace and quiet from your busy mind and begin to think positively.

I hope having this book as your companion will help guide you through your adventure. I'm with you all the way. Amazing things will happen.

Izzy x

Happy

1

Happy ever after

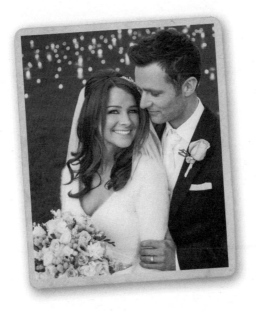

B Y THE TIME Harry Judd proposed to me, we'd been together for just over seven years. We first met in 2005, when I was playing the violin in the backing orchestra on McFly's *Wonderland* tour. By the end of that tour he and I were a couple. When Harry asked me to marry him in the spring of 2012, I'd left the band I was a member of, an electric string quartet called Escala, and Harry had recently won *Strictly Come Dancing*.

The *Strictly* experience was magical for both of us. It was an intense but wonderful twelve weeks during which I saw him change and grow as a person. It wasn't always easy – watching him dance so passionately and intimately with a professional dancer was difficult, and many of my friends couldn't understand why I'd agreed that he should do it! But I understood there needed to be chemistry. I trusted Harry and he never gave me any reason to feel vulnerable.

The admiration I had for him was huge — he put so much work into the competition. Each week, in just a few days, he had to learn things that the professionals had been doing for years, then find the courage to go out and perform to a TV audience of millions.

He and his partner, Aliona, won, as I knew they would. Harry is one of those infuriating people who is good at everything. He's a gifted sportsman — particularly at cricket — as well as a musician, and learns new things quickly and easily. Plus, he has so much confidence and is a born performer. (I'm biased, of course.)

Straight after winning, Harry went on tour with *Strictly* until March and then, almost immediately, back on tour with McFly. Just before he left the second time, Harry told me he'd booked us a spa break in the UK for a weekend in May, so that we could spend some much needed time together, to rest and relax after a frantic few months.

The day before we were due to go, he confessed. 'Actually, we're not going on a spa weekend. We're going to St Lucia. It was going to be a surprise but I'm telling you because I know you'll want to get organized.' He knows how much I like to plan and prepare for everything.

That afternoon, as I was walking down the High Road where we live, I thought, 'Surely he's going to pop the question? Why else would we be going to St Lucia?' I felt incredibly excited. I loved Harry so much, and there had never been any doubt in my mind that he was the person I wanted to spend my life with. We were ready to settle down, get married and start a family.

By the time we arrived in St Lucia, we'd been travelling for nearly fifteen hours and were really tired. I thought it was unlikely that Harry would propose when we were both feeling so jet lagged, so that evening I didn't make too much of an effort – I put on a very simple black dress, even though I'd brought lots of prettier ones, and I didn't bother to wash my hair. While we were in our room I realized how hungry I was, so asked Harry if we could go for dinner. 'Why don't we dance?' he said. That totally took me by surprise but I thought it was romantic too.

So there we were in the room, dancing – to what I don't recall – and I remember thinking it was lovely, but also feeling really hungry and wanting to go for dinner. All of a sudden, there was a knock on the door and a friendly young woman appeared. 'My name's Frances and I'll be your waitress for the evening,' she said, which struck me as a coincidence as my granny's name is Frances.

Frances escorted us to the beach, where a table for two was laid, close to the water's edge. 'Don't Worry Baby' by

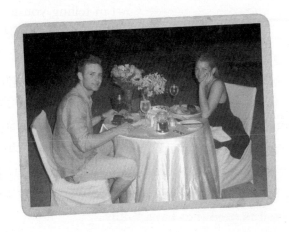

the Beach Boys, a song both Harry and I love, was playing in the background. I'd say it was all of about ten seconds before Harry was down on one knee in the sand! I don't think he could hold off any longer. 'Will you marry me?' he asked, and of course I said yes! We were meant to be together for the rest of our lives, and that was all I ever wanted for the two of us. I was just so happy. I even forgot to look at the ring, which he'd put so much thought into choosing.

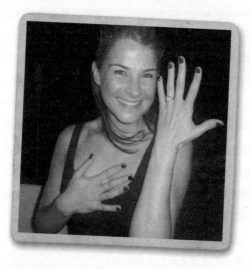

We had a lovely meal, went back to our room, and Harry fell straight asleep. I think he was just relieved to have got the proposal over with! I spent the whole night awake, waiting for it to be morning in the UK so that I could ring family and friends to tell them. But it turned out that Harry had already told everybody before we'd left. There was absolutely no one I could surprise with the news – not my parents, his parents, nor any of our friends. He'd been just too excited to keep it to himself.

Happy ever after

The next day I began writing lists. We planned to get married on 21 December later that year, at St Michael's Manor in St Albans, close to where I grew up. We both thought a Christmas wedding would be magical and neither of us could see any reason to wait very long. We were ready to be Mr and Mrs Judd.

I did all the organizing and Harry did nothing, and that was fine. Planning has always been something I've enjoyed, right back to the days of school projects (I'm totally Monica from *Friends*). As a professional violinist, I'd played at endless weddings with the string quartets I'd been in over the years, so I'd had lots of opportunities to see different ways of doing things, and to think about what I wanted. I loved every minute of making the arrangements and took great pride in getting every detail right. The invitations, the flowers, the decorations, the place names, the music – every single thing was thought through carefully and chosen because we loved it and it meant something special to us.

One of the features I was inspired to recreate was a wishing tree – an idea I'd seen on Pinterest – where guests write their wishes for us on pieces of card and hang them on the branches of a small tree. Much later, during a very difficult time, I took those wishes out from under the stairs at home, where we'd stored them, and read them for the first time. Somehow, I'd never found the opportunity to do so until then, and they were a great comfort to me.

Right up to the last minute, I was coming up with new ideas and finding ways to incorporate them into our day. The night before the wedding we went out for a family meal,

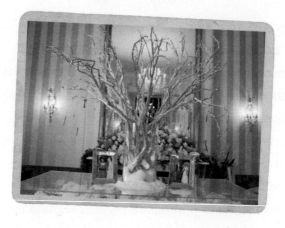

The wishing tree from our wedding day.

and a barbershop quartet were singing in the pub where we were. I asked them if they happened to be free the following day, which they were, and so they came and sang at the wedding reception. It was a risky thing to do, because I didn't have time to ask Harry. Even though he didn't do any of the planning, he liked to have everything run by him!

As Harry was the reigning *Strictly Come Dancing* champion, we had to plan our first dance carefully – we couldn't get away with just shuffling around the dance floor. In the *Strictly* final he'd danced the American Smooth to 'Can't Help Falling In Love', and as soon as I saw him perform, I knew that was the song I wanted us to dance to together on our wedding day. We asked Ian Waite, one of the professional dancers from the show, to teach us. I loved spending time together learning the routine, even though I had to wear anti-sickness wristbands because it involved a great deal of spinning and made me feel so dizzy.

The day was just such a happy one. Full of joy, family,

friends – everything I'd ever wanted. Harry and I were totally sober because neither of us drinks alcohol, but everyone else was merrily drunk. This made the silent disco – where people hear the music through wireless headphones rather than over a speaker system, and you don't need to worry about breaking any noise curfews – even more entertaining, especially when my brother Guy, who'd enjoyed the day a little too much, decided that dancing in his pants was a good idea.

Hello! magazine photographed the whole wedding, and because they'd followed our story from the engagement, it felt on the day like they were our friends, and so discreet and lovely.

One of the best pieces of pre-wedding advice I was given was to have the day filmed as well as photographed, which we did. There's something about seeing the reactions on our family and friends' faces in real time that is just so precious. Sometimes, when I'm at home in the evening, if Harry's out and I'm feeling a bit anxious, I put the film on. It calms me down because it's so happy and takes me right back to that time. All over again, I feel the joy of the day, the warmth and good wishes from the people around us, the excitement and fun we had, and the overwhelming love between Harry and me.

After the wedding, we stayed with our families for Christmas and then, in January, went for a very short honeymoon in the Cotswolds – after all, we'd had a big holiday in St Lucia the previous year.

My life hadn't been a fairy tale up until that point – far from it, as you'll find out. The engagement and wedding to the man of my dreams were so beautiful, so perfect, that I believed my future would be too. And in that idealized future, my first wish was to start a family as soon as possible. I was about to turn twenty-nine and was ready for the next phase of my life to begin.

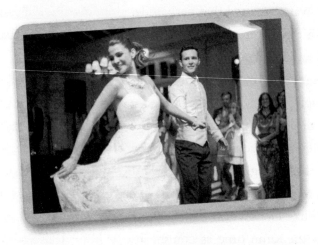

I wanted children, and had done for such a long time. I guess I'm a little old-fashioned but I've always pictured myself as a mum and felt that it's what I'm here to do, the greatest job I could ever wish for.

It never once occurred to me that it wouldn't happen. I just presumed it would, and I couldn't wait. My friends around me were getting married and having babies, and I thought, 'I've found the person I love, we're married, now it's our turn.' Harry was slower to come to the idea of starting a family. Being slightly younger than me he didn't feel the same urgency, and many of his friends were in relationships but not married. I guess he felt we had plenty of time and there was no rush.

I was determined to do everything right. I'd been on the Pill since I was fifteen – our family doctor had prescribed it because my periods were very painful. About a year before the wedding, already thinking about trying for a baby, I sought medical advice about how and when to stop taking it. It was suggested that perhaps by stopping the Pill sooner rather than later, my natural cycle would be given a chance to reset itself.

I came off the Pill shortly after that conversation and sure enough I began getting periods again straight away. For the first three or four months they were heavy and painful, just as they had been when I was fourteen. After a few more months, though, they became much lighter, lasting just a couple of days but still arriving every twenty-eight to thirty days, like clockwork.

At the same time as coming off the Pill, I also stopped taking a drug called Spironolactone. Amongst other things, it's used to treat acne, but you're advised to stop taking it if you're thinking about getting pregnant. Right through my teenage years I had terrible skin but never did anything about it. Finally, though, in my mid-twenties, I got fed up with having spots and went to see a dermatologist, who, as well as prescribing Spironolactone, recommended that I have an ultrasound scan to check for polycystic ovaries – I learned then that acne can be a symptom of Polycystic Ovarian Syndrome. I had none of the other symptoms of PCOS, though – the classic ones tend to be excess facial hair and weight gain, and I'd never suffered from either of those. But I went for the scan and had some blood tests done to check various hormone levels, and found out that I did indeed have PCOS.

The gynaecologist who talked me through the results never mentioned that PCOS is often linked to fertility problems, and that I might have trouble conceiving. I didn't understand the connection until years later when another gynaecologist spelled out the implications for me. Back then, though, I wasn't thinking about pregnancy, I was only concerned about my skin, which cleared up completely once I started taking Spironolactone.

In May 2013 – almost exactly a year since the engagement – with the Pill hormones and Spironolactone fully out of my system, Harry and I finally decided to really start trying for a baby. The instant Harry gave the green light, I was firing ahead, full steam. This was it! I was so excited. I began taking a folic acid supplement and downloaded an app to my phone that told me where I was in my cycle, when I should be having sex and what I should be looking for to tell me if I was in a fertile phase – things like changes in cervical mucus. I was obsessed immediately. I also downloaded another app that enables you to calculate, once you fall pregnant, your due date. I was projecting ahead, madly willing myself into the future I wanted.

Around the same time as we began trying, Harry and I went to Portugal on a seven-day Jason Vale juicing retreat. I wanted to give my system a thorough cleanse because I felt that it would be beneficial generally, and so that I would be in the best shape possible when I fell pregnant.

The week after we got back from Portugal I missed my

period for the first time ever. The date came and went with no sign of it. We were certain I was pregnant. My period was never late, we'd been trying – this was it, I knew it. It all made perfect sense. Our happy-ever-after was about to begin.

I bought a pregnancy test and once I'd done it, Harry got his phone ready to take a picture as I read the result. We thought it would be special to capture the moment, and planned to send the photo to our families. We were both so sure. I really cringe thinking about that now.

But the test came up negative. No second line.

That was fine, we decided. It was just too soon to have taken it. I went online – the beginning of many years of frantic, confused googling – and found plenty of sites to tell me that in very early pregnancy, levels of the hormone hCG (human chorionic gonadotropin) aren't always strong enough to be detected by a pregnancy test.

So, while we waited a couple of days, I did some more research on the internet. I was sure I had some of the telltale pregnancy signs: I was going to the loo more, I definitely felt crampy and bloated. (Of course, I know now that early pregnancy symptoms are very similar to those you get when your period's about to start.) Also, I'd had some blood spotting a week after I thought I'd ovulated, which I assumed, after even more googling, was implantation bleeding. (I later found out it was due to a drop in progesterone. Usually, progesterone levels start to fall just before you get your period. When it happens mid-cycle, it tends to be due to an imbalance of hormones symptomatic of PCOS.)

Harry and I were both still in a state of excitement – I was so certain I was pregnant that already I was being careful about what I was eating and drinking, and how much exercise I was doing. We did another test. Still no second line. A few days later, a third test – and finally, many tests later, I had to accept that I wasn't pregnant.

But I still hadn't had my period. By now I was over a week overdue, having never been late before. I panicked. I completely and thoroughly panicked. I gave myself no time to reflect, no grace period to 'wait and see', no space. Instead, I immediately went into frantic 'fix' mode.

I made up my mind. I was determined to fall pregnant the following month. It was as if, as soon as I'd taken on the idea of being pregnant in my head, I couldn't rest until I was. I needed it to happen – now. I know how unreasonable and impatient that must sound, but it's the way I felt.

I had to get some answers to what was going on, and I didn't even bother going to my GP first. I went straight to the gynaecologist, the same doctor I'd seen to get advice about stopping taking the Pill. He took me seriously straight away. There was no telling me to take a deep breath, give myself a few more months of trying naturally, taking it easy and seeing what happened. He knew my medical history and that I wanted a family, and so decided to get on and find out more.

He did a series of blood tests and scans, and it became clear that I wasn't ovulating. Yes, my periods had always been as regular as clockwork but I now knew they hadn't been true bleeds because I didn't have a 'proper' cycle. This typically happens with PCOS – even though the ovaries contain lots of follicles, the follicles don't develop and mature properly, so no egg is released. Hormone levels then begin to fall and your period starts, even though ovulation hasn't occurred.

Once I found that out, I was in despair. I couldn't believe this was happening. The irony is that, as younger women, many of us go out of our way not to get pregnant and then the moment we start trying, it becomes the hardest thing on earth. I felt completely desperate. I don't remember feeling upset or sorry for myself. Instead, I was frustrated and angry. With myself and with my body. I thought not only was it letting me down, but Harry too. In my head, responsibility for both our futures lay with me, and I wanted to fix the problem straight away. I felt an urgency and a lot of quiet, undoubtedly irrational, guilt.

That missed period was the beginning of a long, hard journey. For me, it was when everything started to go wrong. I felt as if I was completely at fault. When something bad happens, you look to explain it in any way you can and for something or someone to blame, so I blamed myself.

I launched myself straight into a world of medical intervention. Consultations, more blood tests, scans, injections and anxious waits; bitter cycles of hope and disappointment that anyone who has ever struggled to conceive will understand, finally followed by IVF. Much of that time was miserable and some of it was heartbreaking. For a while, I lost myself as a person completely, and Harry and I were tested fully as a couple. But I learned so much: about myself, my body, my mind, my relationship, and what I'm capable of. I learned about fertility, about the process of IVF and how to support it, and about the ways in which the body and mind work together.

With the benefit of hindsight, I believe now that I reacted with too much urgency. I understand why – the thing I had always wanted for myself, a family, suddenly looked as if it might never be, and I couldn't help but throw myself into pursuing that dream with all my energy. I wonder what would have happened if someone had put a hand on my shoulder and said, 'Take a deep breath, Izzy. Slow down. Give yourself a break.' If I could go back in time, I'd tell myself to take a few months to give my cycle a chance to reset itself naturally. Even if it hadn't, slowing down a little would have helped me to confront what came next with more resilience and positivity.

Don't get me wrong, there are, of course, certain circumstances when it's wise to act quickly – when time is of the essence, for instance – and I recognize that I was fortunate enough to see a gynaecologist privately and not have to wait for a referral. But to anyone else who is in the same position now, my advice is: Pause. Breathe. Gather yourself and give yourself a chance to focus. Don't panic. Take it slowly and trust – in yourself and what can happen.

2

A musical family

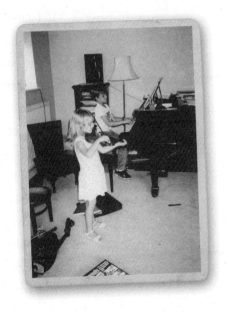

CHILDHOOD SHOULD be a time of wonder for everyone, and it certainly was for me. I was surrounded by a loving family, and what felt like music everywhere. When I look back, it was such a happy time.

My dad was born in Belfast and would have loved to become a professional clarinettist. His father was principal clarinet in the BBC Northern Ireland Light Orchestra and a clarinet teacher, but for his own reasons didn't feel it was the right career for his son. Perhaps he thought it was too uncertain a way to make a living, or maybe he wanted more for Dad. Either way, he refused to tutor him, and so my dad ended up teaching himself. His love for music was just too great to be ignored. He used to listen through the wall when his father was giving lessons to students, and tried to copy what he heard. In the end my grandfather gave in and taught him to play.

Later, my dad moved to London and it was thanks to music that he met my mum. It was 1974 and they'd both arrived late to a music course at Hurstpierpoint College in West Sussex. They began chatting after parking their cars and the rest, as they say, is history!

Mum played the bassoon, and once she and my dad married they set up a music school, Musicale, in Harpenden, the town in Hertfordshire where I grew up. Not only has my parents' passion for music had a huge impact on my three brothers and me over the years but it's also influenced all the children who've passed through their school.

Music has always been what our whole family does, both individually and together. Even Christmas is all about music. Every Boxing Day, as far back as I can remember, my parents would get out the score for Schubert's 'String Quintet' for all of us to play along to, or try to get through as best we could. This was so normal for me, I assumed it's what everybody did on Boxing Day.

We weren't made to play, music was just an organic part of our lives. It was how we entertained, celebrated, even communicated with each other. More than anything, music has always meant home to me because it's something we've always shared as a family. Two of my older brothers, Guy and Magnus, both play professionally, and Magnus is married to a musician. And of course I'm married to a musician too.

In the same way that some people can get lost in a really good book, I can get lost in music, pop as well as classical. I can listen to a piece of music and the years will just fall away, taking me right back to a particular moment in time.

A musical family

When I play, it helps me to express emotion, and when I listen, it helps me to feel emotion at a deeper level than talking ever can. For me, music is the thing that connects me with the world. Throughout my struggle to conceive, during the very hard times, music was such a source of comfort to me. In fact, there is certain music that is so firmly associated with that part of my life that I can't listen to it without being overcome with emotion.

One of my earliest memories is wanting to play the violin, just like my brother Magnus. So for my fourth birthday, Mum and Dad got me a tiny violin. I think my parents realized how lucky my brothers and I are – all four of us have musical ability – and they ensured we made the most of it. They gave each of us the same opportunities, but with music, as with so many things, it's not just about talent, it's about your mental strength – the level of discipline you have, how you cope with the pressure, how much you want to work at it. We each responded differently to those factors.

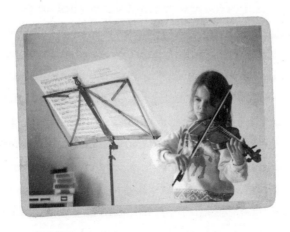

Dare to dream

The effort my parents put into giving us a musical education meant that we earned scholarships to schools they wouldn't have been able to afford to send us to. Rupert, Magnus and Guy all sang in the choir at King's College in Cambridge and went to boarding school there. After King's, Rupert got a scholarship to Wells Cathedral School in Somerset, then Magnus and Guy went to Chetham's School of Music in Manchester. So from the time I was six, none of my brothers lived at home any more. Even though each left in turn and I knew their departure was coming, I also knew what it was like when they did go – a little bit quieter, a bit more lonely each time. It wasn't a sudden change, but I missed having my brothers around me very much.

We were all close, but Guy and I especially so because he's just two and a half years older than me. He was always my buddy (our nickname growing up was Darby and Joan) and I was devastated when he left – all of a sudden it was just me at home. I became very close to my mum and dad – and I adored my granny – but your parents aren't your siblings. The bond between brothers and sisters is very unique.

With the boys gone, life settled into a routine that was busy, despite the house being quiet without them. My days were filled. From the age of about seven or eight, I would get up in the morning and do an hour's violin practice before school. When I came home, I did another hour before my homework, every day. Then, twice a week, my dad would drive me from school into London for my violin lesson, and in the evenings I studied dance and drama. I

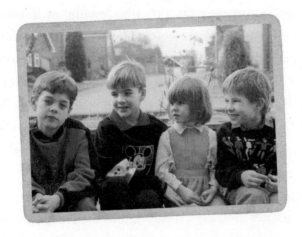

*Me and my big brothers (from left to right)
Rupert, Magnus and Guy.*

loved the arts in general, not just music, and went to both
the Sylvia Young and the Royal Ballet's summer schools.
If there was a stage, I was happy – I suppose I was just a
show-off.

I loved being in my bedroom, and the fact that it was my
space – I was definitely a singing-in-front-of-the-mirror-
with-a-hairbrush type of girl – but I hated sleeping there.
For as far back as I can remember, I've always been scared to
be on my own at night. I need someone to be with me, and
that was another reason I was so upset when the boys left
home – I'd been used to sharing a bedroom with whichever
one of them would have me.

I've always had quite a wild imagination, and it often runs
away with me. I can easily find myself in a different world
that is very vivid, which can be wonderful or frightening
depending on what's in that imaginary world. I don't

remember having nightmares as a child but I never slept very well, waking often and feeling very scared.

I still don't understand the reasons for my fear. I was a happy child and came from a secure and loving family. I've tried tracing it back to something specific without any luck. When I went to a CBT therapist, some years ago, they really wanted me to identify a particular moment or a thing that happened, but there's nothing I can remember that sparked the fear, other than it just being me and that I didn't like being alone.

I remember not ever wanting it to be bedtime. I hated the feeling that the world had gone to sleep and that I was all on my own, with everything shut down and quiet — it felt as if life had stopped. If I woke up and it was light outside, I was fine. But if I woke up in the dark, I was petrified. It wasn't the dark itself, it was being in a world that was unconscious.

Once someone else was in the bedroom, I was fine, whether they were asleep or awake, as long as they were there. (I think that's why I've always liked having a cat at the end of the bed. As children, we had two, my beloved George and Polly, and I still find now there's something comforting about the weight of a cat on the bed and the sound of it purring in the dark.) But if I was going through a particularly bad patch of anxiety as I sometimes did — I had good phases and bad phases — and even if I was sleeping in with one of my brothers, whichever of them was still there, my parents' bedroom door would have to be open. To me, there was a huge psychological difference between an open door and a closed one.

A musical family

Once the boys were all gone, my mum and dad let me sleep in their room on a camp bed for quite a while. Mum had grown up at a time when no lights were left on at night and the house had no heating upstairs, so it was cold, dark and lonely. I think she was probably slightly scarred by that. So if I woke up crying, or if I didn't want to stay in my room by myself, she never forced me to.

My parents also got some advice about my sleeping problems from a child psychologist they knew, who said just to let me sleep in with them until I got over it. I don't know if that was the right thing to say – there are surely better ways of helping children feel comfortable in their rooms by themselves? I'm certainly very conscious of the fact that I want Lola to feel confident sleeping on her own. Perhaps if our lives hadn't taken the turn they did, that advice might have proved correct and I might simply have grown out of my fears.

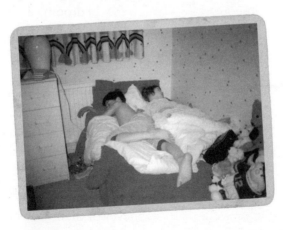

*I had a fear of sleeping on my own as a child,
so would often move in with one of my brothers. On this
occasion, Rupert was my chosen companion!*

Dare to dream

When I got to around ten or eleven years old, I badly wanted to be able to sleep on my own. I was embarrassed to still be in with my parents so I would try to sleep in my bedroom, but more often than not ended up back in theirs, too frightened to be alone. When I was twelve, I began to settle at last. Mum had bought me a TV for my room that could be programmed to switch itself off after a certain amount of time, and I would leave it on while I fell asleep. There was something soothing about the sound of it, low in the background, and I managed a good few weeks of sleeping alone in my own bed.

And then everything changed.

3

The darkest of days

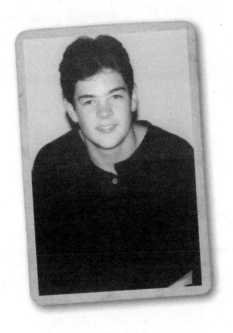

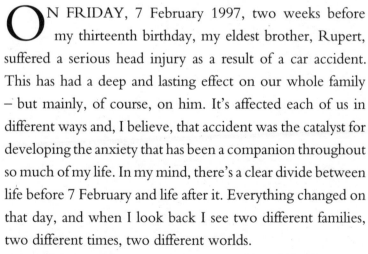

ON FRIDAY, 7 February 1997, two weeks before my thirteenth birthday, my eldest brother, Rupert, suffered a serious head injury as a result of a car accident. This has had a deep and lasting effect on our whole family – but mainly, of course, on him. It's affected each of us in different ways and, I believe, that accident was the catalyst for developing the anxiety that has been a companion throughout so much of my life. In my mind, there's a clear divide between life before 7 February and life after it. Everything changed on that day, and when I look back I see two different families, two different times, two different worlds.

Rupert was eighteen and studying at the Guildhall School of Music in London. He was wild and charismatic, very like my mum in character. Bright, talented, energetic and full of life, everyone at school knew who Rupert was. He was popular, but not always for the right reasons. If something bad happened, Rupert often got the blame, even if it wasn't him, and he'd often take the blame, even if it wasn't him. He was vivacious and confident, and you either loved him or hated him. Half his teachers thought he was an amazing life force, the other half thought he was arrogant and needed taking down a peg or two. I know my mum used to dread going to his parent–teacher meetings and the arrival of his school reports, because the comment was always 'could do better'.

I remember him flying in and out of the house. He never stayed for long as he always had plans – something he wanted to do, somewhere he needed to be. It was Rupert who gave me my nickname of Izzy. My real name is Brittany but when I was young my mum used to say a little rhyme to me: 'Izzy wizzy, let's get busy.' Rupert couldn't say Brittany, so he picked up on Izzy, and it stuck.

Rupert had a real gift for music. He played the French horn and, unlike the rest of us, barely needed to practise – he was a complete natural, which must have been frustrating for some, and had such great performance skills. Even now, there are people who heard him play when he was still very young, back before the accident, who remember something remarkable about what he was able to do.

He began playing with the National Youth Orchestra when he was fifteen, which is extraordinary as the NYO is very hard to get into, especially for brass players. Spaces are limited and only the most talented make it. Magnus still talks about Rupert playing a big Bruckner symphony as part of the NYO. He had this incredible solo and Magnus says it was the moment everybody was waiting for – the whole room didn't move for as long as Rupert played. He was a unique and very special musician.

The night of his accident, Rupert had been out with friends in London but had left early, even though his mates tried to persuade him to stay. He was home by around 10 p.m., but came up with the idea that he was going to drive to Wells, his old school in Somerset, that night – two and a half hours away. One of our cousins, whom Rupert was close to, was in sixth form there at the time. It was just the kind of crazy thing Rupert liked to do.

He told Steve, a friend of his who was living with us at the time – the way many people did over the years – of his plan, and Mum overheard him. She was in bed but often kept an ear open for Rupert's comings and goings. It was already nearly 11 p.m. by then so Mum got up and told him, 'Rupert, you can't possibly drive to Wells.' Of course Rupert reassured her that he hadn't really meant it and was only going around the corner to see a friend. Mum went back to bed then, and to sleep. But tragically, Rupert didn't only go around the corner.

He had his own car, an old white Citroën bought with a bit of money inherited from my grandfather, and he drove all the way to Somerset in it that night. It must have been after 1 a.m. by the time he arrived. He saw my cousin for an hour or so and then said he was heading back home to Harpenden. He refused to stay and get some sleep because, he said, he had a horn lesson at the Guildhall later that day.

Many days later, in the midst of the most devastating

time of our lives, we learned that Rupert's music teacher had rung and left a message on his phone to say the lesson was cancelled. But Rupert's phone was out of battery and he never got the message. We listened to that voicemail afterwards, and that was one of the hardest things – knowing there had been no reason for Rupert to leave Wells that night. He could have stayed. He could have been safe. All of our lives could have been different.

There are so many 'what ifs' and 'if onlys', but we would send ourselves mad if we thought too hard about them.

From what we know, Rupert left Wells at about 3 a.m., and he got to the junction joining the M25 and the M1 sometime around 5 a.m., at which stage he was only about ten minutes from home. The exit is a stone's throw from where he crashed. He so nearly made it.

He drove into the back of an articulated lorry. We think he probably fell asleep at the wheel but we'll never know. He could have been fiddling with his stereo, or reaching for something. His car went underneath the lorry and was torn up like a tin can. The M25 was shut; fire engines, police cars and ambulances arrived. Rupert had to be cut out of the wrecked car. He was dead at the scene and only brought back to life by a defibrillator. It's a miracle that he survived but we've sometimes asked ourselves whether his survival was a good thing. It's a terrible question to ask, but with everything that followed, I think my parents have thought, at times, that perhaps it would have been kinder, given Rupert's quality of life now, if the tragedy had begun and ended that morning on the M25.

For Mum and Dad, the first they knew about the way in which all our lives had changed was when the doorbell rang very early in the morning, when all of us should have been in the house and safe asleep. At first, my dad thought it was Rupert, and that he'd forgotten his keys. When he saw the police, again his thoughts went straight to Rupert. Dad assumed Rupert had done something and was in trouble. But when the officers quoted the car registration number, asking Dad if Rupert was the owner of the vehicle, Dad knew instantly that something was terribly wrong and he fell to the floor in a state of shock.

My mother's first reaction was to say that she hoped Rupert hadn't broken his arm, because he was due to play in a concert at King's the following evening with my other brothers.

I remember the moment I heard about the accident so clearly. I'd slept in my own room that night, and early in the morning Mum opened my bedroom door to let me know what had happened. She explained that she and Dad had to go to the hospital and I'd have to get myself off to school. I remember hoping Rupert hadn't hurt himself too badly, but not being too alarmed. In fact, those were probably the last innocent thoughts of a young teenager who knew nothing about loss or grief. I had no idea how much our lives were about to change. I just went back to sleep until my alarm went off and it was time to get up as normal.

Mum and Dad were driven to the hospital by the police, who were unable to tell them much about what had happened, or even how Rupert was. Steve, Rupert's friend, was at home so I wasn't alone, and we just presumed at that stage that Rupert was going to be OK. About an hour after my parents had left – it was still very early and I hadn't yet gone to school – the phone rang. It was Mum, letting me know that a police car was coming to fetch me and take me to the hospital. I grabbed Rupert's beloved Snoopy teddy, as I hoped it would cheer him up. I imagined him sitting up in a hospital bed, getting better from his accident, with Snoopy keeping him company.

When I got to the hospital, Mum and Dad were sat in a tiny, dreary family room, their chairs pulled close to each other for support and their shoulders hunched. Seeing them there, I immediately understood that something was very wrong. I'd never seen them looking like that before – the emptiness in their eyes and fear in their voices was terrifying. It was as if my pillars of strength had crumbled. They weren't crying – I think they either didn't dare allow themselves to, or were perhaps in too much shock – but it was as if they weren't quite there. I remember trying to take it all in but feeling completely lost and frightened. I just wanted to go home and then to school, where life would be normal. I wanted what already felt like a terrible nightmare to end.

Mum and Dad hadn't even seen Rupert at that point – the nurses had advised them not to go in because of how very badly he was injured. The head injuries he'd suffered were catastrophic and he was on life support. So they'd just been sitting in that room, passing the phone back and forth between them, ringing various people to tell them the terrible news. Neither of them could really complete a sentence, so they took it in turns to try to deliver the information, which they barely understood themselves, to family and friends.

Instinctively I wanted to help, so being upset wasn't an option in my mind. I wanted to do something to fix things, to make them feel better, and the only thing I could think of was to offer to fetch them tea and coffee.

I remember a nurse coming in and saying, 'We're going to wheel Rupert past.' They were moving him to a different hospital called Atkinson Morley, in Wimbledon, which specialized in neurology and neuroscience. I wanted so much to see him, but the nurse said it was best I didn't because he was too ill. So I asked her to give him the Snoopy, because I wanted him to have something from home.

Since the day I was born, I've had a Winnie-the-Pooh bear that has always been such a comfort to me, and I hoped Snoopy would be the same for Roops that day. The nurse was very kind and said she would give it to him, but really I wanted to do it myself. I remember being so confused as to why I couldn't see him, and when I handed Rupert's Snoopy over to the nurse, I suddenly wanted it back; I realized it had been comforting me.

For all the strangeness of the hospital, I only really began to understand how very bad things were once we got home and I started to pick up on the atmosphere of fear. Even though I was thinking about Rupert, I was more sensitive to what I could see around me, and that was Mum, Dad, Magnus, Guy and my granny. I was very tuned in to them and their reactions. I was certainly being protected from the full story, but I had an intuition that I wasn't being told everything.

I remember being sat on my granny's knee and asking her if Rupert died whether he'd be with my grandfather. The thought of him going to heaven gave me comfort, as I knew he'd be safe there. My granny was the real matriarch of the family, and she and I were very close. She was the anchor, the person who held it all together. She'd been through so much herself – the war, losing her husband, siblings and friends – and she was so strong that she gave me hope that everything would be OK.

About a week after the accident, during which time Rupert remained on life support in the intensive care unit, he had brain surgery – a twelve-hour operation followed by every conceivable type of setback. First he contracted MRSA. Then one of his lungs collapsed. Then he got pneumonia, followed by a cranial fluid leak, which meant more surgery and a tracheotomy – which is where they make an incision in the windpipe to relieve an obstruction to breathing. But Rupert is such a fighter.

He contracted pneumonia on my thirteenth birthday. I'd been looking forward to this birthday so much – I think any girl's thirteenth is exciting. I was having a disco with friends in the hall of my parents' music school. However, before the party got under way, Mum told me that Rupert was unwell and they had to go back to the hospital. The party still went ahead but without my parents there. I remember feeling irritated that they'd gone, that I couldn't even have just this one day. Perhaps because Mum and Dad tried so hard to make sure life went on as normal for me, I wasn't fully aware of just how bad things were.

The first time I saw Rupert after the accident he was still in intensive care, wired up to so many machines, which he hated – they had to put the blood-pressure monitor on his toe instead of his finger because he kept tearing it off. I remember the ICU so clearly – it was somehow peaceful, despite the near-constant beeps from the machines. Sometimes, in between the noises, I could even hear the clock ticking on the wall behind the nurses station.

The other patients around Rupert were also in very serious conditions. I was both too young and too old to cope well with that; too old not to understand what was happening, but not yet old enough to comprehend the full implications. I so badly wanted to do something, anything, to help and to make people feel better, but there was little I could do.

When tragedy happens, the world seems to stop, but soon enough a normal kind of life resumes. The trauma doesn't go away, so you learn to live around it. At a certain point, those who have visited with food and flowers have to go back to their own lives but you're still left with a terrible new reality. That's when you know – really know – who your true friends are, because they're still with you. And we were lucky. We had many true friends.

The doctors couldn't tell us much immediately after the surgery, as at that stage they had no idea exactly how much damage had been done. The hope was that the parts of Rupert's brain that hadn't been injured would gradually learn to take over the functions of those that had been, and that Rupert would start to re-learn any skills he'd lost. They told us this could take up to ten years.

At first Rupert wasn't able to communicate at all. The tracheotomy meant that he couldn't talk, and there were very few other signs of response from him. The only real sign of life, or memory, came through his reaction to the classical horn music we played to him. One day we even gave him his French horn to hold. He couldn't play it, of course, but he started to move his fingers in time to the music. That was the first indication we had that he recognized something, that somewhere in there the Rupert we knew was trying to communicate with us.

In the months following his operation, progress was evident every day. He slowly started to learn to walk, to talk and to feed himself again. But it got to a point, about a year later, once he'd re-learned these basic life skills, that it became a question of seeing how much more he was going to improve, and what his permanent cognitive injuries would be. Today, twenty years down the line, we're definitely at a point where we know there won't be any further recovery. For a long time, we were watching every day, desperately hoping, but then I think we slowly began to realize that he wasn't going to get any better than he was. Although the realization was gradual, it was very painful.

We'd hoped for a miracle – that Rupert would return fully to himself. Beginning to accept that that wouldn't happen meant saying goodbye to the Rupert we had known, and mourning the person he could have been. It's still something we experience every day. I don't think we'll ever fully come to terms with it.

For many months, Rupert's bed stayed exactly as I had found it on that first morning, because Mum couldn't bear to go into his room. The room continued to smell of Lynx Africa, and his Charles Worthington shampoo stayed in the bathroom, even though no one else ever used it. For a long time, we expected him to come home, and so everything stayed right where he'd left it, waiting for him.

Although Rupert did come home briefly after his long stay in hospital, my parents quickly realized that they couldn't cope with him living there. It was a difficult time as we were all in a state of confusion about Rupert's needs and how best to look after him day to day. Eventually, after much thought and advice from local services, it was decided that it would be best for Rupert to move to a residential home

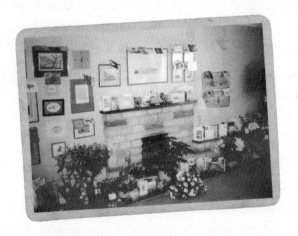

*Our home after the accident, covered in
cards and flowers.*

for rehabilitation and ongoing care. I can only imagine now what a heart-wrenching decision that was for my parents to have made.

Today, Roops is basically an exaggerated version of the person he was before the accident. You never forget meeting him! He walks into a room and people are immediately aware of his presence. His behaviour is very friendly and he's immensely loving and giving, but he can often be inappropriate because he has no awareness of boundaries or personal space. He'll sometimes shout at the top of his voice in crowded places, or get up and begin walking around when it's not appropriate to. He can't settle to any occupation for very long and constantly wants to know what's happening next. He lives in either the past or the future, but finds it difficult to be in the moment.

What's almost more frustrating is the fact that he is so nearly there. He's capable physically, engaging, understands nearly everything and knows who everyone is. He can still play music beautifully and take part in conversation. There's just something missing, a layer of awareness. He's childlike, but in an adult's body, with adult language, adult strength and some adult knowledge.

He's also very conscious of what he doesn't have. Major life events have a profound emotional effect on him because he understands that they may never happen for him – he's unlikely ever to get engaged or married or have a family, and he's deeply saddened by this. As are all of us, for him.

When I accepted Harry's proposal, I felt so guilty when I thought about Rupert. I'm so lucky to have Harry and it seemed incredibly unfair that Roops may never experience the same feelings of love and happiness, as he's such a warm and loving person himself. In so many ways, Rupert's life stopped the day of his accident.

Mum was very worried about how Rupert would behave on our wedding day. She was concerned that he would be disruptive in some way, such as coming up to the altar during the service. There had been discussions about him being there just for the ceremony, missing the reception and returning for the evening celebrations, but I insisted that he stay for the whole day. I didn't mind if he was disruptive – as far as I was concerned, he was welcome to stand with Harry and me throughout the whole ceremony if he wanted to. I wanted to make him feel it was his celebration as much as mine. 'After all,' I thought, 'if he can't be himself on my wedding day, when can Rupert just be Rupert?' And he was brilliant. He played his French horn during the service, and of course made the most of his moment, coming out and taking a bow before the congregation. Then, during the after-dinner speeches, he was even heckling with one-liners, making everyone laugh.

But it was very hard too, for all of us, because even though Rupert was happy for me, and happy to be there, he was terribly emotional. My brothers Magnus and Guy played as I walked down the aisle – 'Gabriel's Oboe' from the film *The Mission* – and in the recording, on the wedding video, you can clearly hear Rupert sobbing. I can't listen to it without wanting to cry for him.

Rupert has so much to offer but we all still grieve for

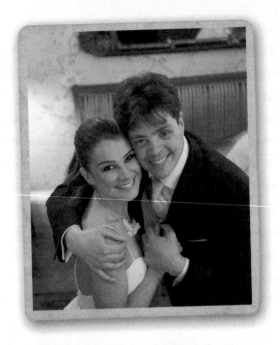

*I wanted Roops to feel a part of
our wedding celebrations.*

what we've lost. His music career, which was so promising, tragically never materialized. He requires twenty-four-hour care, can't lead an independent life and never will. We love the person who is here now, of course we do – he's our brother, my parents' son – but it's impossible not to wonder sometimes about what he might have been had this never happened.

That was the reason I later set up the Eyes Alight appeal, to raise money for victims of brain injury. To try to give Roops back a little something of what he had lost. And because my way of dealing with the sad and terrible things that sometimes happen is to try to make something good come out of them. It's the same impulse that later made me want to be honest about my IVF experiences – the idea that I could help others, and that the hard times I went through could somehow be turned into something positive.

Twenty years ago, my family's life changed for ever. I'll remember every second of 7 February 1997 for the rest of my life. It is through tragedy that you discover so much about yourself and others. It changes the way you look at life. You learn who will stay by your side to help you through the difficult times. There's a handful of truly special friends to Rupert, the ones who still visit, answer his endless phone calls and brighten up his day. These people are amazing and I don't think they realize what their kindness means to my family and, of course, to Rupert. Harry has become a best friend to him – he loves him unconditionally and that's just so special. He reminds me to take Rupert for who he is today – a unique, inspirational and awesome brother. I couldn't imagine my life without Rupert in it.

Through my darkest times when my anxiety was unbearable and my desperation for a baby was taking over my life, somehow Roops always seemed to be sitting on my shoulder, reminding me to keep things in perspective and try my hardest to make the most of each day. This isn't always easy, of course, but I've tried my best. I feel I owe that to him and the fight he put up for life. But most importantly, Rupert has taught me to celebrate life, family, friends, love and everything we have to live for.

4

Shockwaves

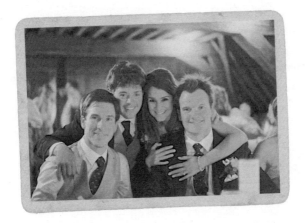

RUPERT'S ACCIDENT brought us much closer together as a family; however, individually it affected each of us in different ways. For my parents, caring for Rupert took precedence over everything else, whether they wanted it to or not. Once my mum began to understand the new realities of Rupert's life she became far more accepting of them. For my dad, it was harder to let go, and I think he still feels that accepting the changes means somehow giving up on Rupert. Magnus, who had always had his older brother, suddenly felt a weight of expectation to step into that role, and Guy lost the person he had always looked up to.

For me, Rupert's accident and the terrible change in our family life brought huge sadness, which has never gone away. That sense that I never really got to know my brother as I should have done has always stayed with me. The theft of his life as it should have been has always been very hard to contemplate.

Even now, I can't drive on the stretch of the M25 where Rupert had his accident without shivering, and without my thoughts keeping pace with what happened to him: 'Rupert was fine up to this point. Still fine. Still fine.' And then, suddenly, '*Bang!* Everything changed here.' The accident happened beneath a bridge and every time I drive under it, I find myself thinking, 'How is it possible? Up to here, he's fine, and then a metre later his life just stopped?'

If I'm listening to the radio and hear there's been an accident close to where anyone I care about lives, I have to ring them and make sure they're OK, and if anyone I love goes on a long car journey, I always need to know that they've arrived safely.

I think it's evident that the accident brought about a huge surge in anxiety for me. If I'd gone through a more natural process of growing up, I'm sure I would have developed in confidence and overcome my fears. But when a tragic accident happens in your family, you develop a sudden understanding of the stark realities of life and death: the implications, the danger, the possibilities of awful things happening. When I look back, it seems to me that I skipped a significant part of normal teenage development. I became an adult very suddenly, but with no emotional maturity.

This meant that throughout my teenage years, any time I had a struggle or a concern, I never felt it was 'big' enough to allow myself to express it, because it was always so much smaller than what had happened to Rupert. For me, that was the natural thing to do, not a conscious decision. So I kept all of my worries to myself and didn't tell my family what I was going through.

Following the accident, I began to find that I couldn't switch off. I couldn't let myself relax, because if I did I wouldn't be in control and something bad might happen. I had a fear that if I fell asleep I wouldn't wake up, that if I stopped minding myself and let myself go, I might just disappear.

These feelings became the root of my anxiety, which became my close companion. I've taken to calling it 'my friend' because it's with me constantly and because, ultimately, I've found it more helpful to think about it that way than as an enemy. It's still a part of my life, even now, although I manage it far better these days.

As well as myself, I began to worry about the people around me, in particular my parents. I wasn't able to fall asleep until I knew they were in bed sound asleep and safe. I just felt such an enormous sense of responsibility; in my mind, I had to keep the show on the road and so I felt I had to be alert at all times, in case something happened. At first, my anxiety was mainly confined to night time. I could fall asleep without too much difficulty but shortly afterwards would wake again in a panic. I'd sit bolt upright instantly, shaking with fear, in a state of complete terror. I felt as if there was a lion in my face, ready to attack me; something immediate and life-threatening, except I never had a name for what it was. I think an actual lion might have been easier to deal with, because what I had was fear of the unknown, fear of the future, fear of what might and could happen.

I didn't hyperventilate, as I know some people do. For me, panic manifested itself as the icy grip of fear, and the effect of that fear was very physical. I would often spend most of the night on the loo with an upset stomach, and my legs would shake uncontrollably. It's a surge in adrenaline that causes this: adrenaline is the fight-or-flight hormone and once it's released the body gets ready to fight for survival or run away. Lots of things happen on a physical level to make you hyper-aware and reactive – including your heart rate increasing, your pupils dilating, tunnel vision and shaking. But when there isn't any actual physical danger the sensations are very uncomfortable and, for me, frightening. It becomes a fear of the fear, something I understand a lot more now, but back then I didn't, I just knew how bad I felt.

There were nights when the anxiety would come and go for four or five hours; other nights it lasted just half an hour or so. When it passed, I would feel such relief, as if my body was being bathed in a calm, warm feeling – that's the endorphin release, after the intensity of the fear – and I would fall back asleep. But it was exhausting, physically as well as emotionally.

Once morning came, I could busy myself and try to push the panic out of my mind. I would get on with what I had to do – school, music and homework – but always, underneath it all, I knew that it would be night time again before long, and that once it came I would experience the fear all over again.

After a while, the panic attacks began to leak into the daytime, specifically triggered by any kind of change. If I ever had to go away – for a school trip, or a music course – I became very nervous and didn't want to go. Over the years, the fear worsened, reaching a peak when I was with Escala and often had to gig overseas, usually on very short notice.

I never really spoke to anyone about Rupert – about what had happened and the way I felt about it – until eventually, a good few years after the accident, a friend's aunt who was trained as a therapist asked me out of the goodness of her heart to come and have tea and biscuits, and to have a chat to her. She's a beautifully intuitive person and could see I needed to talk.

At first I found it very difficult to actually say anything, to express myself at all, but when I did finally start to talk about it, it was as if the room went black. Suddenly I felt I was back at the time of the accident. Something unlocked inside me and I told her things I didn't even know I felt. It was wonderful to let it all out – the sense of relief was overwhelming – but once was enough. I never really spoke about it again. Perhaps I should have, but I didn't see the point of going over and over the pain and the trauma.

I found my own way of dealing with worry and anxiety, and that was to remain in control. At the age I was, all you really have the power to control is yourself. So I chose not to drink, for example, and I still don't. I can count on one hand the number of times I've had a few, and I can remember clearly how awful I felt afterwards. Also, being drunk means you're out of control, and I hate that. I never seemed to get nicely tipsy like other people do. I tend to bypass that stage and get quite fiery. Alcohol just doesn't go with my character. I never liked it, or what it could do to me. I still don't like the way it can change someone's personality.

As part of my need for control, I'd plan what I had to do very carefully, even obsessively. I didn't make any spontaneous decisions and, as far as possible, I didn't travel. I kept as tight a rein on everything in my life as I possibly could. Even so, there would be occasions when the anxiety gripped me so hard I couldn't sleep, or concentrate. I certainly couldn't shake it off.

In my mind, this anxiety had a profound impact when it came to wanting to start a family. What happened to Rupert gave me a craving to have my own family; there was something about it that felt like a fresh start. I thought that grandchildren would be another chapter for my parents, too; something to look forward to. For Rupert as well, as he's unlikely to have children of his own, a baby would mean the chance to be an uncle. So as much as I wanted a child for my own and Harry's sake, I also felt that bringing new life into the world would be a really positive thing for my family.

For all the wanting and craving, I think my long struggle with anxiety had something to do with the fact that it didn't happen naturally, and it also contributed to my PCOS diagnosis. When it comes to fertility, if you're constantly in an anxious state, or worried, or in that heightened fight-or-flight mode, your body doesn't naturally do what it needs to do to reproduce. Looking back, I feel I was trapped in a vicious circle. Women with PCOS are thought to have higher levels of anxiety and depression than those without.

When you're under stress for long periods, the body releases hormones such as adrenaline and cortisol into the bloodstream. Without getting too scientific (I'm no doctor), this plays complete havoc with your hormone balance and is therefore believed to contribute to the symptoms of PCOS.

I believe that my body was telling me that it wasn't safe for me to be pregnant because I'd essentially spent ten years living in a heightened state of anxiety, keeping myself in check all the time, which takes a huge toll, physically and mentally. It was so frustrating to hear other people telling me that I just needed to relax. If only it were that simple! Even though I did everything I could think of to calm my anxieties and conceive naturally, I believe now that my body simply wasn't able to let go of the tension. And probably, the more I wanted it and the harder I longed for it, the less likely it was to happen.

5

Feel the fear

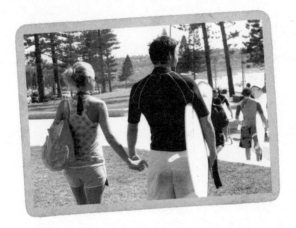

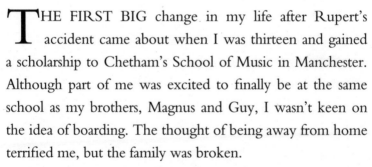

THE FIRST BIG change in my life after Rupert's accident came about when I was thirteen and gained a scholarship to Chetham's School of Music in Manchester. Although part of me was excited to finally be at the same school as my brothers, Magnus and Guy, I wasn't keen on the idea of boarding. The thought of being away from home terrified me, but the family was broken.

Rupert's needs were so great that my parents and I decided it was best for me to join Magnus and Guy at Chetham's. It would provide me with stability and focus, and, musically speaking, a fantastic education. Although I didn't love being away from home, I was mostly happy there, and the change was a positive thing.

It wasn't that I was ever unhappy exactly, more that I was grieving – for Rupert, for my parents, and for the fact that we'd lost our family as we'd known it. That colours my memories of my time there but there were a lot of good things about Chetham's. I had a fun year group, and because I shared a bedroom with three other girls, I don't remember my anxiety being that bad, despite feeling homesick. I went home for the weekend every three weeks and was very much in touch with Mum and Dad in between – I had a little pager, and they would send me messages: 'Call home. Mum.'

Throughout my time at Chetham's, I suffered from chronic period pains. I can remember times when I was bent double, as the pain was so intense. When it was particularly bad, I had to go to sick bay for the day with a hot-water bottle for comfort. The nurse gave me painkillers and let me lie down, but no one ever suggested that something might be wrong and need investigation, even though it happened every month. Going through that kind of thing when you're young and away from home is embarrassing, so it didn't cross my mind to talk to anyone about it in more detail. It was only when I got my period at home once, when I was about fifteen, that Mum asked, 'Is this what it's always like for you?' When I said yes, she took me to the doctor, who put me on the Pill as it's known to help with painful periods. Even then, there was no real investigation into why the pain was so bad.

A few weeks into my final year at Chetham's I began to have serious doubts about my future as a musician. I'd started to lose my passion for playing the violin, and so my parents suggested that I come back home, finish my

A Levels at my local school and have a break from the intensity of music school. I carried on taking violin lessons with the most inspiring teacher, Howard Davis, and he completely rekindled my love for music. As a result I decided to audition to continue my studies with him at the Royal Academy of Music in London and gained a full scholarship.

During my first year there my mum spotted an ad for a violinist to join a new all-girl classical-pop crossover group. Although I'd fallen in love with music again, I was still confused about what I wanted to do exactly – I wasn't certain about carrying on studying classical violin. I missed drama, dance and performing generally, and I also felt the need to do something a little different to my brothers; to carve out some space just for me. There would be far more performance involved in a group, more need for the sort of stage engagement I missed from drama and dance.

So I auditioned for the group and in 2004 got the part in a five-piece called Wild, created by the same management that had started Bond, the all-girl quartet who had formed in 2000. They'd gone on to have huge success all over the world and while Wild weren't as successful, we had a lot of fun and I learned a lot about the industry. We released an album, *Time*, and played lots of corporate gigs in Australia and Asia. Best of all, some of us went on to form Escala.

Even though Wild only lasted a couple of years, the experience changed my life. I began to play the electric violin – a big jump for a classical musician – and that became my career. It was also through Wild that I met Harry (albeit indirectly) and my best friend, Chantal. Chunny and I instantly forged a lovely friendship that has been a source of such strength to me ever since – she's like the sister I never had. I've often felt as if she and I go through many of the same things in our lives, the same difficulties and upheavals, although with her slightly ahead of me, like my guardian angel. I feel very lucky to have found a friend who loves and supports me no matter what and who always has time to really listen. She's the kind of friend you can cry with, sit in silence with for hours without it feeling awkward, and who you can laugh just that little bit harder with (she has the most infectious laugh – it's impossible not to join in!). She is someone I would feel truly lost without.

Even though I was enjoying myself with Wild, I still suffered from a great deal of anxiety when it came to travelling. I began to realize how little I liked existing in a world where I could be told at a moment's notice that I might be flying to Asia for a gig. I had, up until that point, managed my anxiety by trying always to be in control, but it soon dawned on me that the career I had launched myself into wasn't compatible with that.

After a couple of years, Wild began to fizzle out. We could all feel it – the excitement wasn't there any more, and I think we were all ready to move on. At that time Chantal and I were asked to go on tour with a band called McFly, as backing musicians on their *Wonderland* tour. Initially, because of contractual obligations, we had to say no but we managed to sort things out eventually so that we could take the job. It became one of those *Sliding Doors* moments: while on the *Wonderland* tour Chantal and I met the other

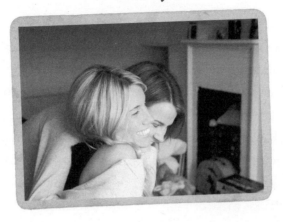

Chantal's like the sister I never had.

members of Escala – Victoria Lyon and Tasya Hodges – and I
met Harry. I got a new career and a boyfriend, all in one go!

We formed Escala with Vicky and Tasya because we
found that we loved playing together – there was real
chemistry and friendship between the four of us. We began
to gig and recorded an album, then, in 2007, we performed
at the *X Factor* wrap party. It was there that the producers
of *Britain's Got Talent* saw us and invited us to audition for
the show. It was a little bit controversial at the time because
we were professional musicians and some people felt that
wasn't fair. The controversy never bothered me as the show
is open to everyone, amateur or professional, and in a funny
way it's more of a gamble if you're professional, because you
have more to lose. None of us had a day job to go back to –
music was our job – so we knew we had to nail it.

I remember the audition stage in front of the judges so
well. We waited all day to play for them, and got so nervous.
We'd had to sit backstage in these little purple dresses for

hours – there wasn't the right sound equipment, so we couldn't go on. When we finally did, it was amazing. We got a standing ovation from the audience, Simon said we were 'incredible' and Amanda called us 'phenomenal'. We were used to performing in the background at parties, weddings, launches, with people talking, laughing and having drinks while we played. So it was a whole new, wonderful feeling to be in the limelight. But for me, the wonder didn't last.

Harry and I were a couple by that time, I was teaching violin and had been gigging with Escala at a level I enjoyed. I was happy and liked my life, which had a simplicity to it – I knew what I was doing from day to day, what hours I was teaching, where I needed to go. As a freelance musician, you're either free to accept a gig, or not. It's that simple. You have control over what you do, and don't need to answer to anyone except yourself. And when you're with someone like Harry, whose profession is so unpredictable, it can be hard, but we'd found a rhythm. Now it was all about to change.

Once Escala got through to the semi-finals of *BGT* and things began to take off, any control I had vanished completely. As part of a group with a manager, agents and band members, you can't just say yes or no. You have to go where you're told, do what you're told. There's very little that is certain and I hated that. I was afraid of my life changing, because I was so happy with how things were.

Before the semi-finals, I thought it would be a good distraction from my worries to go to Australia with Harry, where McFly were recording their album *Radioactive*. In fact, it was the exact opposite of a good distraction because, while there, I had the worst panic attack I'd ever experienced.

It was a beautiful day and the sun was beating down from a clear blue Australian sky. I was sitting on a vast white beach curved like a horseshoe. Harry was off surfing, so I set up camp with my book and my music. I was alone, the beach was quiet and quite empty, and I was absolutely fine reading, when all of a sudden I felt completely disorientated. I was afraid to stand up I felt so dizzy.

I immediately wanted Harry but he was so far out in the water I could barely see him – I certainly couldn't wave to him or attract his attention. He'd only been gone about ten minutes, which meant he wouldn't be coming back any time soon – he'd usually be out surfing for up to an hour. When you're having a panic attack every second seems like an eternity, so the idea of waiting so long for him to return was unbearable.

Because I felt so dizzy and out of myself it crossed my mind that I might have been suffering from sunstroke, so I realized I needed to get out of the sun. I felt as if I had no control over my body or the sensations going through me. What I felt was fear so strong that it had become an incredibly physical sensation. I thought I was going to die or that I'd never come back to myself, that I would continue to float, lost, outside my body for ever, unable to reconnect with it. I wanted to go home so badly but home was 10,000 miles away.

I finally managed to stand up and make my way to the car, every few minutes thinking I was going to fall over. I got in, shut the door and reclined the seat so that I could huddle down and stay out of the sun as much as possible. I kept trying to steady myself but the waves of fear just continued to come over me. Eventually I rang my mum back in England and spoke to her. Hearing her voice comforted and reassured me, but the call must have been distressing for her. She knew I had panic attacks, of course, but I'd be in my room at night when they happened and I'd deliberately kept the full extent of them from her. She never knew how bad they could be until that moment.

Time passed horribly slowly. After a while I saw a girl I knew, so I jumped out of the car and ran after her, begging her to find Harry for me. He was back on the beach, so she went and got him. The minute he was with me I started to calm down.

That was far from the end of it, though. When you have an attack like that, you're so afraid of it happening again that the anticipation becomes almost as bad as the attack itself. That evening, I became very upset at the thought that my anxiety had taken on a terrifying new form and had spilled out from where I'd been able to contain it and into the rest of my life. What happened down on the beach had been different to the night-time attacks. It wasn't remotely normal for it to happen in the middle of the day out of nowhere.

I became too worried to enjoy the rest of the trip. I couldn't control everything happening around me, obviously, so I controlled the only thing I could, and made sure I was never on my own. Being alone made me feel physically sick with fear.

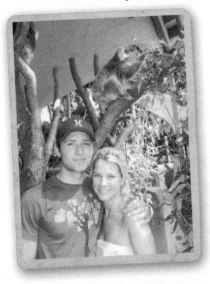

*I suffered my worst ever panic attack during
this trip to Australia.*

Once back from Australia, things got so bad that I couldn't
even get into the shower unless Harry or my mum was in
the bathroom with me. Even then I had a constant feeling
of dread hanging over me. I felt that Escala was wrecking
my life, ruining my relationship, and yet I felt utterly torn
because I knew I was so lucky to be a part of this amazing
opportunity. I was so angry that anxiety was holding me back.

By the time Escala played in the final of *Britain's Got
Talent*, I was in a miserable state. In order to go on stage
that night I had to take a Diazepam, and when I watch the
footage now it's clear how terrified I was – I can see it in
my eyes when the judges are critiquing our performance.
I'm sure no one else noticed, let alone had a clue what was
going on, which makes me realize how easy it is to look at

other people and presume that they're absolutely fine – or better than fine, perfect even – when in reality we have no idea what's happening with them.

That night should have been wonderful – the judges told us we were world class – but instead I just wanted it all to stop, to go away. The sad thing is that I wanted to want it. There I was, standing on the threshold of what had once been my dream, and I hated it. The conflict was huge. I knew it was the anxiety that was stopping me, holding me back, so I was tortured with wondering, 'Am I going to give in to anxiety, or am I going to fight it? And if I decide to fight it, can I even do that? How can I possibly win?'

Immediately after the final, the *Britain's Got Talent* tour started. By then, I was in such a state that I wasn't even enjoying the actual performing – I felt very frightened on stage and it had just become a case of getting through each performance. The other girls knew, and they were so kind about it, but really, there's only so much anyone can take of someone being as demanding and needy as I was. They were young, excited, about to launch into this amazing career, and my emotional state was tough for them to handle.

I lost myself completely. I went from being a competent, capable, confident person, to being dependent, hopeless and childlike. The lowest point of all came one day when we had a show in Newcastle. Mum and Dad had driven for five hours to take me there, but when we arrived at the hotel I refused to get out of the car. Instead, I insisted that we go home. They talked to me, calmed me down, and somehow I managed to get into the hotel. We sat on the balcony outside our room overlooking the Tyne Bridge and I remember reflecting on how bad things were, and wondered what my life was becoming.

As well as being a particularly low moment, it was also perhaps a turning point for me. Although I'd been through talking therapy as well as taking medication by this point, and I could just about function, I wasn't happy at all. I was in a constant state of anxiety and the only relief from it came when I fell asleep. Fortunately, and somewhat ironically, somehow I *was* able to sleep – I imagine because I was so tense all day, I exhausted myself.

Soon after that trip to Newcastle, my mum decided that enough was enough and took a much tougher approach with me. This is something I'm very grateful for now, but at first I was angry and defensive. However, once I thought about it I saw she was right, and from that moment, bit by bit, I started working to get out of that terrible place.

I began to properly do the exercises I'd been given by the CBT therapist I'd seen. They were based around the idea of growing comfortable with some of the sensations the anxiety produced in me, and included having to spin around – to get used to feeling dizzy and to know that the feeling was OK. I used to find bright light really uncomfortable because all my senses were heightened and my pupils dilated, so another exercise was to stare into a light until I acclimatized. I'd also have to go to a supermarket, because I found them really overwhelming, and would practise being on my own in one aisle while Mum was in another, then meeting her at the end.

At first, I'd done these exercises half-heartedly, and only because I like to please. They made me feel uncomfortable and embarrassed. Being twenty-one years old and unable to function as an adult was humiliating. But I began to throw myself into them a bit more, and they did help.

Somehow I fought the anxiety and stayed with Escala but it was exhausting. We performed, toured and gigged, and while it was very difficult, I did it and I'm glad that I did. But the travelling never got easier. Every time I had to go away, I'd think of ways I could lose my passport or miss the plane. Chantal would have to hold my hand from start to finish. It was like babysitting, and bless her for doing it.

Anxiety is much worse when jet lag is involved because you end up tired and eating strange food at weird times. Fatigue and blood sugar levels both have a lot to do with anxiety because they're related to adrenaline: low blood sugar causes the body to produce extra adrenaline and that in turn will cause the kinds of symptoms – a racing heart, dilated pupils, shaking – that I found so uncomfortable.

On top of this, the adrenaline and stress hormones flying around the body wreak havoc with the endocrine and, in turn, reproductive systems – as I've mentioned, there's a known link between high anxiety levels and PCOS in women. It's no coincidence, I think, that good nutrition to control blood sugar levels can help with symptoms of PCOS as well as anxiety. Back then I think I was stuck in a vicious circle. These days, I understand it all so much more clearly and therefore I can help to manage my symptoms better.

As I've said, I now look on anxiety as my friend rather

than my enemy. I have to, because I've learned that it's something that will always be with me in some shape or form – it's a part of who I am. I can't get rid of it so I have to live with it as best I can. This has meant learning to manage it, because fighting it doesn't work and leaves me feeling worse. I eventually found mindfulness, which has made a big difference to my life – and is something I'll talk more about later – but it took me a long time to get there.

Through this time Harry was always supportive and I never felt any pressure from him. He just said, 'Don't do it if you don't want to. Just leave the band, Izzy, if that's what you want.' I knew Harry was always on my side no matter what I decided to do, because he always had been, from the first time we met.

6

All about Harry

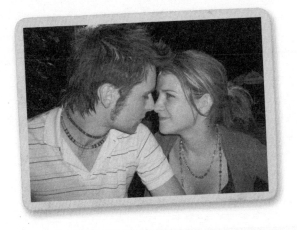

I'VE ALWAYS FELT that my granny – my mum's mum – sent me Harry. She and I were so close, and she died the summer I met him. She was ninety-four and had been the solid centre point, the rock, of my life. When I lost her, I lost a lot. I missed her terribly, and still do. I feel her presence in my life even now, and there have been times when I was suffering the most, when I have felt it more strongly.

The summer of 2005, when I met Harry on McFly's *Wonderland* tour, was a funny time for me. I didn't know a whole lot about McFly, although I did own one of their records. I'd heard 'Obviously', their second single, on the radio and liked it, and I remember going to WH Smith in Harpenden to buy the album, *Room On The 3rd Floor*. I know I thought some of it was quite up tempo – with heavier drumbeats than the pop ballads I was used to, anyway – which makes Harry and I both laugh now, because it's far from heavy! But I didn't know one band member from another, or anything about them as people, I just liked their music.

Before the tour started, the guys were doing an interview on TV, and Mum called me in to watch it. She pointed out Harry as he'd been to Uppingham School – which Magnus had also attended for a while before he went to Chetham's. I didn't think anything of it at the time, of course.

At that point, I'd been going out with Rupert's best friend for five years. We'd known each other for ever, and he'd also lived with us for a while after Rupert's accident. Early that summer he'd ended the relationship, so by the time the McFly tour came around I was broken-hearted as well as grieving for my granny. I certainly wasn't looking for a new boyfriend.

And yet the first time Harry came into one of our rehearsals I felt something so strong for him. I'll never forget seeing him and feeling instantly that I knew him, that I'd known him for ever. We were in a church in Bristol, rehearsing for the band's *Wonderland* tour. The orchestra was in place, tuning up, when in walked the band.

They all came over to say hello and when Harry introduced himself to me, I went red. Chantal thought this was funny because just hours earlier I'd been crying over my ex-boyfriend and now I was blushing over Harry! I kept thinking to myself that this wasn't the plan, to fall for someone else, but it happened and just like that Harry was in my life. I tried to tell myself it was nonsense, that it couldn't be true, that he was a nineteen-year-old pop star who probably had five girlfriends, and for professional reasons I shouldn't get involved. But I really liked him – I couldn't help myself.

Then, as luck would have it, two days later I got mumps and was sent home. My parents were away on holiday, my brothers were busy working, and I was ill, alone and utterly miserable.

I rejoined the tour two weeks later and spent the next few weeks feeling as if I was in primary school all over again. Every time I saw Harry I got embarrassed, to the point where I avoided him, hiding whenever he came along. The thing was, he felt the same way. He remembers meeting me that first day in the church and saying to one of his bandmates, Dougie, that he fancied me. When he turned up a couple of days later for another rehearsal and was told one of the girls had had to take time off because of mumps, his immediate thought was, 'Please don't let it be Izzy.'

McFly's management weren't keen on the band hanging out with the orchestra out of working hours. They were probably worried we might be a distraction, so there weren't many opportunities for Harry and me to see each other except for at the arenas and on stage during the gigs. At that time I smoked, as did Harry, and he'd often knock on the girls' dressing-room door and ask if anyone wanted to join him outside for a cigarette. He says he only did it to see me, and remembers wondering why I was never there. In fact I was, but hiding behind the door or in the loo, too embarrassed to come out. We also later discovered that each evening before the show we'd both walk around backstage, hoping to bump into each other, but somehow we never did unless it was in catering when there were too many other people around.

McFly's big hit at the time was 'All About You', and every night on stage when they played it, Harry would turn to hit the tambourine, which was right in my eye line, and would look at me. And I would look at him. Even that got awkward, though, because each show I'd wonder if he was going to look or not, and then felt embarrassed for thinking about it so much. We talk about it now and it's funny but at the time it was utterly cringy. I fancied him madly but didn't know what to say or do. One of the other orchestra members, Dave, knew how I felt, and he told me it was mutual, but you don't believe that unless the guy himself says it to you.

On the penultimate night of the tour, in Cardiff, there was a party. It was the first time we were formally allowed to socialize with the band after hours. I remember Harry politely speaking to everyone in the orchestra except me. Finally, he came over and said hi, and offered to buy me a drink. I ordered a soft drink of course, and he said, 'Are you sure you don't want anything else?' I explained that I didn't drink, and later he told me that at that point he thought, 'Damn, I can't even get her drunk.'

We chatted for a long time and as we talked I found that I could be myself completely. There was no pretence, no trying to impress, no faking anything. I knew straight away that Harry and I spoke the same language. I felt that I understood everything about him – all the important things, anyway. That feeling I'd had the first time we met – that I knew him, had always known him – only got stronger. I think we told each other things that night that neither of us had spoken about much to anyone else. It just felt so easy to open up to him. He made me feel like no one else had ever done before. He was interested in everything I had to say and really listened. I felt safe and happy around him, like nothing else mattered. Most of the others went off to a club, but we went back to the hotel bar with a few people and continued chatting for hours. I told him a bit about why I didn't drink, about my family, my parents, Rupert.

Then Harry went out into the lobby and the next thing I knew, one of the band's security guys came in and asked if I'd come outside for a minute because someone needed to talk to me. I was really worried that I'd done something wrong, but it was Harry. He wanted to get me on my own but didn't want to ask in front of everyone else in case he embarrassed me – or himself if I said no! We went outside then and had our first kiss, and really, that was it for both of us. It was magical, as if the world stopped for a moment. I knew then that Harry was going to be in my life. There was something about him that felt magnetic.

I had a few last commitments with Wild before things wound down – we had three weeks of performances to do in Australia soon after the McFly tour – so I went off to do that, which was probably a good thing for Harry and me. I'd just gone through a break-up and a bereavement, and tour life is notorious for being heightened and intense at the best

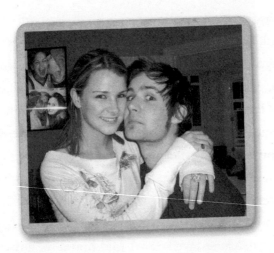

of times. You're in a bubble and at the end of it you need to come down and figure out what's real.

I spent the whole three weeks in Australia looking at photos of Harry, ringing him and thinking about him. He spent the three weeks getting rid of the girlfriends he'd been seeing before he met me!

I never worried about Harry with other girls, only whether he was too young to want to settle down. My attitude towards other girls was simple: if he's going to do it, he's going to do it. I'm not a jealous person and perhaps that was because I was a bit older, and successful in my own right with my own career – I wasn't sitting at home, waiting for him. I also understood the music industry and the way it looks a lot more exciting and glamorous from the outside. I never felt, 'Oh, Harry's famous …' It was just a very normal lifestyle.

Harry's a very sensitive, loyal and compassionate person – I felt that to be true about him from the start. A couple of months into our relationship he met Rupert and that confirmed my instinct. I took Harry to the home in Aylesbury where Rupert lives, then we went for pizza and took Roops bowling – his two favourite things! Harry was amazing. From that day, Roops and Harry became great friends. Rupert adores him, and Harry, in turn, loves Roops and gets on with him brilliantly. At family events, he'll always spend time with Rupert, who can be exhausting company because he's always asking, 'What next? What now?' Harry isn't fazed by that. He enjoys Rupert's company and understands his needs so well. He's become a best friend to Roops and loves him unconditionally. For me, this means everything, and I know my family has been very touched by the amount of compassion he has shown towards Rupert.

Soon after we got together, I told Harry about my anxiety. I'd never have tried to hide it – not that I think I could have. I also felt that it was so much a part of me that Harry would have to either take it or leave it. He has so much warmth and empathy, though, that I felt he'd understand, and he did, even though at first he wasn't aware of how bad it was.

I think he first began to realize the extent of what it was like for me when he saw how much I wanted to be with him every night. At the very beginning, he might have mistaken it for being controlling but actually it was nothing to do with that. I just didn't want to be on my own!

Harry was so good. But for anybody living with someone who has a mental illness – which is what my anxiety is – there can come a point where it all becomes too much, and I know there were times when he found my behaviour challenging. Mental illness can make you selfish and difficult, even when you don't wish to be or don't understand that's what you're being. It's tough to be a carer, even if you love someone. It's draining. You're constantly on call and your life isn't your own.

Happily, a big change came about when I decided to leave Escala in 2012, just before we got married. I left on my terms – because I wanted to and because I knew it was the right moment, not because the anxiety forced me to. The sense of relief at getting back to making my own choices was huge and it enabled Harry and me to feel as though we could move forward with the next chapter of our lives together.

Through all of the difficult times, at the core of our relationship, there has always been a huge amount of understanding and love. Harry and I were attached from day one. I just knew that I wasn't going to go through life without him. I could never picture myself walking down the aisle towards anyone else.

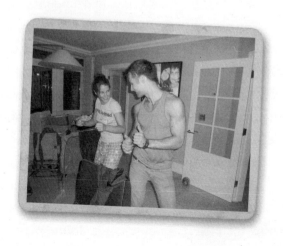

All about Harry

I believe that spending so many years together before getting engaged, and growing up together through our twenties, meant Harry and I really knew and understood each other when we got married. And I'm sure it made a big difference later, when we found ourselves trying to conceive.

My mum always said that there are men you fall in love with and there are men you marry, and that the two are very different. Harry once heard her saying it, and wanted to know what she meant. But I already knew. With Harry, I fell deeply in love, but it's our friendship that has kept us going.

As well as being kind, Harry's always made me laugh. He has a sense of humour about everything. He's much calmer than I am, and willing to go with the flow, which made things feel less awful and serious than they would otherwise have done during the years of trying for a baby. He was able to see us both through the darker days.

7

Losing myself

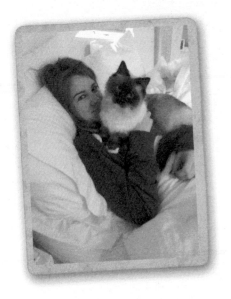

THINKING BACK to my reaction at finding out that I wasn't pregnant after all, following our juicing retreat in Portugal, and the way in which I instantly panicked when the pregnancy test was negative, I can now see so clearly the things I should have done differently. I immediately became obsessed with the idea of being pregnant, and I wonder if that complicated things for me mentally. The pressure I put myself under from that point onwards was intense, and can only have made things worse. I really envy women who are more laid-back and happy to give things time, to see what happens. It just wasn't in my nature to respond calmly – I suppose it stems from my anxiety and, as a result, the desire to be in control. I wanted answers, reasons and reassurance. I needed to understand why I wasn't ovulating, and get it fixed, fast, so that I could get pregnant.

Polycystic Ovarian Syndrome is the most common hormonal disorder among women, affecting about 10 per cent of us, although different women are affected to different degrees. When it comes to ovulation, often what happens is not that you don't produce eggs, you do, but because of an imbalance of hormones, a mature egg isn't always released from its follicle, so you don't always ovulate each month. This then can mean that your ovaries are filled with follicles that have failed to release eggs, which can lead to cysts forming.

PCOS isn't an automatic cause of infertility, though – and this was really important for me to remember. Women with PCOS get pregnant all the time. Some need no assistance at all, some need a little. I never believed that PCOS was the root cause of my problems. I've always thought there was more to my inability to get pregnant, that the amount of stress and pressure I felt from the moment we decided to try for a baby, and even before, had an impact. This belief played a large part in my attitude towards everything that happened to me during the two and a half years between first thinking I'd fallen pregnant effortlessly and finally having Lola.

I believed then, and I still believe now, that my mind played as large a part as my body did in my inability to conceive naturally. At first, this was an entirely negative belief – I blamed myself. I thought that because of my anxiety I wasn't strong enough to be a mother, and that nature somehow knew this so wasn't permitting me to become one. I began thinking this way pretty early on – I've said before how I have quite a wild imagination, which runs away with me a lot. Instantly, I believed it was my fault, not Harry's, and that it was my failure as a woman.

After that first missed period, my cycle never returned, and with that came desperation. All expectation and hope seemed to have been taken from me so quickly. As well as running the hormone tests and scans, which determined that I wasn't ovulating, my gynaecologist also discovered that the lining of my womb was thin. This meant that my chances of getting pregnant naturally at that time were very low, and that I was going to need help and intervention to get my cycle going again.

In September 2013, three months after the Portugal holiday, I was put on a drug called Clomid, to stimulate the ovulation process. For some women, Clomid is a miracle treatment and there are many stories about how successful it can be, but it didn't work for me.

Clomid has plenty of side effects, and as soon as I started taking it – one pill each day for five days, starting on Day Five of your cycle – I began to experience them immediately. I put on weight, suffered from bloating and water retention, and my hormones shifted hugely. It felt as if my body was completely resisting the drug. I became tearful and low, and my skin got really bad, all of which affected my self-esteem. Not everyone responds as dramatically, but for me Clomid had a strong and instantaneous effect. I felt dreadful but I continued to take it because I wanted to be one of the many success stories.

During the first month I was scanned internally throughout

my cycle to monitor my ovaries and check the lining of my womb. The gynaecologist needed to know I was getting the correct dose of the drug – too little and you won't ovulate; too much and you risk over-stimulating the ovaries, meaning you might end up with triplets! But nothing happened. My body was indeed resisting the drug. I was getting the side effects but not ovulating; all the misery with none of the gain. So the following month my gynaecologist upped the dosage. I did ovulate that time, which was encouraging, but I didn't fall pregnant. However, it was a start.

I was then told to continue taking the higher dosage of Clomid for six months. The gynaecologist said he didn't need to see me or scan me now that we knew the drug was working, and that we should all just wait and see what came about. Because I knew I'd ovulated the month before, I felt reasonably OK with this. It seemed positive, as if falling pregnant were just a question of time now, and so I decided that I could put up with the side effects.

Life did change, though. All I could think about was getting pregnant and I tracked each cycle obsessively. I knew more about the inner workings of my body than I could ever have imagined. Harry quickly learned a whole lot about my reproductive system too! I was so in tune with parts of it that previously I'd paid no attention to.

When you're trying for a baby, it feels as if you live your life day by day, month by month, chained to your menstrual cycle. For the first few days after your period, you're waiting to try to conceive. You're then fertile for about five or six days, so you feel you need to be having sex all the time during that window. Then there's the waiting to find out if you're pregnant – two weeks of just getting through the days, killing time before you can do the test. It's awful. It dominates everything, takes over every waking second.

Even during the times when you can't 'do' anything, there's always something to look for or anticipate. Your life doesn't feel like your own, your mind doesn't behave as you're used to. Everything is heightened and you're constantly interrogating your own body: 'Has my temperature gone up?' 'Do I feel crampy?' 'Am I tired?' 'What does it mean? What does it mean? What does it mean …?' I remember saying to a friend how much I wished I could look inside myself and see what was going on with my body. I googled endlessly, looking for symptoms and signs that I might possibly have conceived. In the very early stages of pregnancy almost everything could be a symptom, which is confusing and often misleading.

Sex feels completely different too, and not in a good way. This is something I'm sure all couples who experience fertility issues discover. I think Harry couldn't believe his luck at first, but sadly sex becomes routine and functional very quickly: 'It's Day Ten, we've got to have sex!' 'I'm ovulating, we need to have sex now!' You end up having sex not because you want to, but because you need to, because now is the time you might conceive, so go, go, go! Regardless of what else you're doing, or had planned to do – drop everything! There's an urgency and a clinical quality to it that is so far away from what it should be. Suddenly, there's no fun, no joy, no flirting or romance left – instead, it just becomes routine. You think about what the optimal positions are for conception, how you mustn't go to the loo afterwards but stay lying down with your legs in the air instead. Oh, and then you read something that says having sex too often reduces the sperm's potency ... So then you wonder how often is too often? What's optimum?

On top of all of this, my body was changing physically and I was putting on weight because of the Clomid. I didn't feel attractive or feel like sex – I think even Harry got sick of it all – and yet it was as if we were obliged to.

It must have been hard for Harry, because in this kind of situation men can feel almost used; as if it's not *him* you want, but rather what he can do for you. Luckily, Harry's humour kept us both going. He'd laugh at me for insisting that he mustn't go in the sauna when he went to the gym, because heat is bad for sperm count and motility. He'd come back and I'd say, 'You went in the sauna, didn't you ...?' I'd be cross but he'd tease me a bit, gently, and I'd try to find the funny side.

Then I found a piece of research on the internet that said the chance of conception increases if both partners orgasm together – well, we both giggled about that. As if life wasn't already difficult enough, we were now supposed to add simultaneous orgasms into the mix!

But as much as we tried not to get too caught up in the frustration of trying and failing, at a certain point we both lost our sense of humour for a while. There wasn't a moment I didn't think about getting pregnant, and it wasn't happening. My obsession didn't go as far as thinking about life with a baby, it was just about conceiving. I wondered was I somehow less of a woman if I couldn't get pregnant? I ended up questioning my whole identity.

Despite taking the Clomid, I still had very little faith in my ability to get pregnant, and that meant I had very little faith in myself. In fact, as the months went by and nothing happened, it seemed to me that I was going backwards. That my body was becoming even more reluctant to become pregnant. I grew ever more bloated, I had bad skin, my complexion was pasty. Looking back, I can see that I became depressed. I was reluctant to go out to social events and would say to Harry, 'I don't want to come. I've got nothing to wear that fits me, I don't like the way I look, I've got nothing to talk about. I'd rather stay here with the cats, in my tracksuit bottoms, watching a film …'

I know we're all supposed to be better than this – to have loads of inner resources so that the way we look doesn't matter. But the truth is, it just does. We don't necessarily want to look amazing, we just want to look and feel like ourselves. And I didn't. I felt awful, and I felt that I *looked* awful, which I minded. I've always been someone who eats well, and while I was still exercising during this time, my body wasn't reflecting any of the work I was putting in. I began to wonder what the point of it was. I felt neither energized nor motivated. I was tired and miserable.

I even began to exercise less, thinking, 'I'd better not run in case I'm pregnant. I'd better not lift heavy weights in case I'm pregnant …' Because that was all I wanted to be, and I was so desperately hoping it would happen. The effect of not exercising was that I felt worse. It all became a never-ending, vicious circle.

Anticipating things began to take over my life. I ended up existing, not living. I was no longer in the present, but constantly projecting into the future: 'If I'm pregnant, when will the baby be born?' Every big occasion that happened – Christmas, birthdays, holidays – I was thinking, 'I wonder will I be pregnant this time next year? Will we have a tiny baby by next summer? Where will we go on holiday if we do?' I even remember booking a room at a hotel for a friend's wedding and wondering whether I should book a travel cot. Each month the anticipation was followed by disappointment, and so we stopped making plans.

My life was on pause. I couldn't make any decisions about what to do with myself. I was drifting, waiting, hoping, and feeling more and more miserable with every month that passed and every negative pregnancy test.

The descent into depression happened so quickly. In the space of just a year I went from getting married, deciding we were ready to start a family, going on holiday, thinking I was pregnant and being so happy, to being this strange, bloated, miserable person with no energy and bad skin. I didn't even recognize the person I'd become.

For Harry, life had to go on as normal – and that meant being away often, on tour with the band. And wherever he went, I went too! I'm sure the other guys sometimes thought, 'Go home, Izzy, this isn't very rock 'n' roll with you around.' But when you're trying for a baby, you need to be together, and anyway, I missed Harry. The band would frequently be away for a month at a time, which is a long time not to see someone, especially when you're newly married and want to be together constantly.

Usually, I love life on tour – you stay in lovely hotels, you don't have to cook or clean, and you're in a funny little bubble where you take it easy during the day, then watch the gig at night and hang out backstage. It's fun. But at that time I probably would have been better off at home, given how unsociable I felt. However, being home alone wasn't possible because of my anxiety, and going to stay with Mum and Dad wasn't what I wanted either. I just wanted to be with Harry.

On the McBusted tour in the spring of 2014, Harry's bandmate Tom and his wife Giovanna had just had their baby boy, Buzz. Gi and Buzz came on the tour too, as Buzz was only a few weeks old, and I spent many nights back at the hotel with the two of them. It was just lovely. I'd watch longingly as Gi and Buzz went through their nightly routine. First a bath, then a feed, and then Gi would sing a lullaby before putting Buzz in his cot.

Gi was always a support to me during our struggles, and someone I always felt I could talk to. Even with a tiny newborn she had time to listen, and we shared many moments when I cried on her shoulder. I remember going into her room one night and totally breaking down because I was so miserable, and she just sobbed with me.

I found it hard, socially, whenever people asked what I was up to because to me, life was paused and I couldn't move forwards. I'd left Escala before we got married and only just started my next venture, an online gift store called Izzy's Attic, so I didn't have much to say in response. It was even worse when people asked whether, now that I was married, I wanted children. And people did ask. In fact, those questions started very quickly after the wedding. Surely we all know by now that not everyone finds it easy or possible to have a baby, and we should be sensitive to that? And yet they do ask. It's like the elephant in the room. Sometimes they'll even advise you not to leave it too long, as if you're not making an effort or haven't thought of that yourself!

Because of everything Harry and I went through, if ever I hear of someone who has been married for some time and doesn't have children, I tend to assume they might have

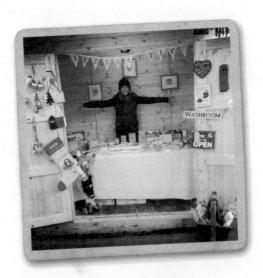

I set up my own gift business called Izzy's Attic but my mind could only focus on starting a family.

struggled, and I wonder briefly what their story might be. It's very possible that they may not want children, but my own experiences lead me to think there's sometimes more to it than that. For that reason I never ask. And I won't talk about Lola unless they do, just in case I'm adding to their pain by doing so. I remember so well the dread I felt when those 'don't you want a baby' questions came up.

I dealt with the situation as best I could by avoiding going out. If I did go out and someone asked, then Harry and I would reply, 'We're practising.' That was our line and thankfully people often would leave it at that.

During the third month of taking Clomid, my period was three days late, and when it did arrive the bleed was really heavy, with a great deal of pain and cramping. I rang my gynaecologist, who said it was nothing to worry about, that it may have been due to ovulating and having a thicker lining than usual, but I still wonder whether it was a very early miscarriage. It was the only indication I had during that time that the drug was doing what it was supposed to do – stimulate ovulation.

After four terrible months and no positive pregnancy test, I went back to my gynaecologist so that he could track my next cycle and, sure enough, as I'd feared, I wasn't ovulating. It was heartbreaking.

So, in January 2014, my gynaecologist took the next step and booked me in for an HSG (hysterosalpingogram), an X-ray of the fallopian tubes when a special dye is injected into the uterine cavity to detect any obstructions blocking the egg from making its way to the uterus. This was followed by a tubal cannulation, which means flushing the tubes to clear any potential blockages, and both procedures can be pretty uncomfortable. For some women it helps clear blockages and can increase their chances of falling pregnant; however, for me, it determined that my fallopian tubes were clear.

They discovered at that stage that I have an unusually shaped cervix, which had made the HSG particularly uncomfortable. My uterus is also retroverted (backwards-tilting) and while this isn't particularly common, it's nothing unusual; it's a bit like being left-handed, apparently. Neither of those things had anything to do with infertility but it was useful to find out, particularly for down the line with IVF.

By this point I was thoroughly fed up and wanted a second opinion. In February 2014 I changed gynaecologist and it was recommended that I try another month of Clomid, but this time alongside a drug called metformin, which can help to manage some symptoms of PCOS. Sadly for me I responded badly to the metformin and experienced terrible nausea. In some people, this side effect can settle over time, but I felt so awful that I was keen to come off it immediately.

I was then referred to a different gynaecologist at the same clinic, Dr Ram Navaratnarajah, who was a specialist in fertility and could help further with assisted conception. A kind, gentle man and wonderful doctor who saw me through everything that followed. He re-ran my hormone blood tests, as a few months had passed since the previous results, and suggested that our next step be something called IUI (intrauterine insemination). This involves first giving medication to encourage the ovaries to produce eggs – a follicle-stimulating hormone called Gonal-F, which has yet more side effects such as headaches, fatigue, and bloating again – followed by an injection of the hormone hCG, to bring about the growth and release of a mature egg. Once the egg is released, sperm is placed directly into the uterus, and this gives a greater chance of fertilization.

I injected the Gonal-F every day for fourteen days, with regular scans to check on the growth of the follicles. By then, I'd watched my ovaries on the monitor so many times, they were nearly as familiar to me as my own face. But nothing happened. The eggs didn't grow, and so there was nothing to release. And because no egg was released, we couldn't complete the IUI. Again, I felt like a total failure. My body continued to resist all our efforts.

Even though he always remained cautious, my wonderful doctor was also positive and encouraging. He showed me the follicles on screen and, to try and cheer me up, told me, 'Look at them all there, waiting. They're having a party. We need to get them to grow, but they're all there!' And that did make me feel a bit better – you have to try to hold on to your sense of humour. But despite his best efforts, I couldn't escape the feeling that we were beginning to run out of options.

All around me, everyone I knew seemed to be getting pregnant. Every time I opened Facebook, there was another announcement. Every time the phone rang, it was a friend wanting to tell me her good news. Or that's what it felt like, anyway. I tried so hard to be happy for them, but each announcement hit me that little bit harder.

Dare to dream

During that time, I could barely walk down the high street – I couldn't stand to see pregnant women or new mums pushing their babies in buggies. If I saw someone shouting at their child, or just being bored by them, or impatient, I couldn't bear it. I'd watch and think, 'You don't know how lucky you are! Why you? Why not me?'

I hated myself for thinking this way. I didn't want to be the person I felt I'd become, with the personality that had been imposed on me by my failure to have a baby.

Around that time a friend who'd got married after me and Harry got in touch to suggest we meet up. She'd sent a message asking how I was, to which I replied honestly

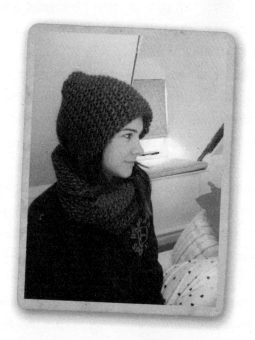

During this terrible time I just wanted to hide away.

that I wasn't great; that I was having a tough time and felt miserable. I wasn't specific about what I was going through, but I thought she might have guessed.

We met for brunch and no sooner had she sat down than she said, 'I've got some news ...' Of course I knew straight away. Sure enough, she was pregnant. Two hours of having to sit and listen to how excited she was, what the scan had been like, which hospital they were going to, the kind of birth she wanted. By the time she asked about me and how I was feeling, I couldn't say a thing. It wouldn't have been appropriate and I don't think I physically could have voiced my troubles.

That was a very low point for me. I wanted to sob, to hide away. Every part of me hated myself even more, because I felt the desperation of trying and failing to get pregnant had destroyed my ability to be happy for a friend. I walked home thinking, 'This is awful. What have I become?'

I called Harry and I cried and cried. I felt so isolated, and angry that it seemed so easy for some people while I was going through hell. I tried not to let it consume me but it was hard not to. I'd even started to think that this might be it, that I might never have a child and that I'd spend the rest of my life unable to handle other people's happy news. It was unbearable. There was no part of me that was prepared to accept it.

At the same time, though, as always, my mind turned to Rupert and I told myself to be grateful: in Harry I had someone to hold me, someone to come home to at night. Rupert is unlikely ever to have that kind of relationship with anyone. I knew that I was lucky and that I should be content. But at the time I couldn't be.

Harry was far calmer than me about what we were going through — not many of his friends were married at that point, let alone involved in the kinds of dilemmas we were facing, and he definitely didn't feel the same urgency that I did. Thank goodness, because one of us needed to stay calm! I felt guilty for failing him, and frightened that I might not be able to give him what I knew he wanted: a family. In the long run, I wondered, was he really going to be OK with that? It's not that I ever thought he would leave, but I worried for his happiness, because I knew he would be such

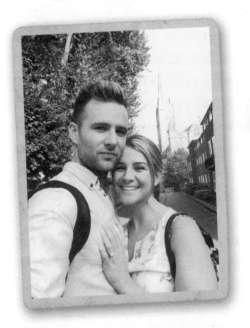

Through the hard months of constant disappointment, Harry was the only person I could really talk to.

a great dad. I worried that he would have to compromise too much in what he wanted. And I worried about whether I was enough for him, if we never had a family. I was scared of how my state of mind might be affecting our relationship.

One day, after yet another negative pregnancy test, I came downstairs and was so sad. There were no tears, I just felt completely empty, exhausted and drained of all joy. Harry got down on his knees and said, 'Izzy, worst case scenario, it's you and me. That's still a pretty good scenario, right?' In that moment I was reminded what an amazing husband I had. Sometimes, you get so lost in a situation that you forget what you do have and how lucky you are. I knew he was right, that it was a good scenario. Even if we never had children, I knew a life with him would be enough to make me happy. That was a huge moment for me, one I'll never forget.

Harry and I were a team. He was the person I could really talk to (or sit happily in silence with), and he never wanted me to feel that everything was on my shoulders; I knew that we were in it together.

After eight months of Clomid, metformin and the failed IUI, I was deeply discouraged. Those months had been hard on my body and hard on my mind. I'd reached a very low point and knew something drastically needed to change.

8

A whole new me

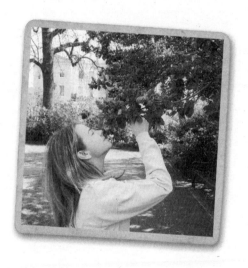

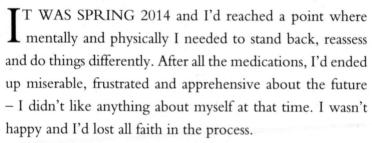

IT WAS SPRING 2014 and I'd reached a point where mentally and physically I needed to stand back, reassess and do things differently. After all the medications, I'd ended up miserable, frustrated and apprehensive about the future – I didn't like anything about myself at that time. I wasn't happy and I'd lost all faith in the process.

There had to be a better way; I needed to make a change. And so I made the decision to stop taking all medication, for a while anyway, and even stop trying to get pregnant until I'd given my body and mind a chance for a complete rest and cleanse. The first thing to do was a complete detox and I really meant complete: mind, body and spirit. Growing up, my mum had always told me to 'make things happen', so I got the bit between my teeth. If things had to change, I was the only one who could make that happen.

Dare to dream

I was determined that I didn't want to be examined, scanned or quizzed for a little while. I was so fed up that mentally, somehow I found I was able to park the idea of getting pregnant. It felt right. In fact, with hindsight, I should have taken this breathing space at the start of the process, before getting in a panic, seeing doctors and agreeing to interventions. Hindsight is a wonderful thing. The past year had been a constant cycle of anticipation and disappointment; of wondering what the future might be, then being heartbroken when it didn't bring what I wanted. I'd been frantic, wearing myself out by watching, waiting, hoping and wondering. Now, I knew I needed to stop it all and say, 'I'm not doing this any more.'

It was May 2014, a year and a half after the wedding. I was thirty years old. I decided to set aside six months and use all of my willpower to get myself into the best shape possible, mentally and physically. My plan was to draw a line under everything that had happened, and go forward with a whole new mindset. At the back of my mind I knew that if I was in optimum health I was more likely to conceive, but my motivation for doing it was not solely that. I wanted to rid my body of all the drugs I'd taken – the Clomid, the metformin, the Gonal-F – because I'd developed a very negative attitude towards them. I hadn't become one of their many success stories. Instead, my body seemed to have resisted them and I'd experienced every side effect going. I felt as if they were still in my system, clogging me up, holding me back and keeping me the unhappy, insecure person I'd become. I'd also begun to consider the way in which my anxious mind was perhaps affecting my body, and knew that it was time to try to enter a calm, relaxed, positive mental state. Easier said than done, but I was going to try my absolute hardest.

I wanted to do it for Harry, too. During our fertility struggles, I sometimes felt like I was neglecting him and our relationship. You become so focused, so obsessed with one thing – getting pregnant – that you forget the person beside you, the person who is on this journey with you. I wanted time to reflect on the good things: the fact that Harry was my world no matter what else happened or didn't happen.

Living a clean, healthy life was within my control. It was something I could do myself – I'd hold the reins and make the decisions – unlike the fertility treatments, which were almost entirely in the hands of my doctors.

I felt excited about what I was going to do, and energized in a way I hadn't been for so long by the prospect of doing something proactive and giving myself a different focus. Several years earlier, I'd begun to look into what causes spikes in adrenaline, because of the effect this has on anxiety. I'd already learned a great deal about the links between sugar and caffeine and the endocrine system, and as a result had reduced my sugar intake and cut out caffeine completely.

I carried on down this road and began to do even more research into diet and fertility – I learned so much from Marilyn Glenville's book *Natural Solutions to PCOS*. When you suffer from PCOS and anxiety it's really important to keep your blood sugar levels steady and some sources I read

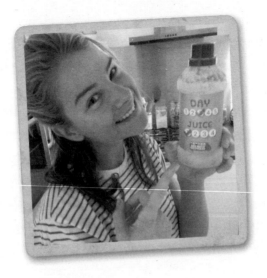

Taking back control – nutrition was a key part of my new approach to my fertility problems.

recommended following a sugar-, dairy- and gluten-free diet to help with this. I began to eat only fresh food that I'd prepared myself, plenty of vegetables and lots of oily fish. This wasn't only to improve my PCOS symptoms (and in turn hopefully my fertility) but also for other health benefits.

I started to take some supplements too – a fertility-support multivitamin, magnesium to boost my reserves and help reduce my body's stress reaction, omegas 3 and 6 to help the quality of my eggs, vitamins D and C because they can help to regulate hormones, and a probiotic to improve my tummy health, especially after all the medications I'd been taking. I wanted to give my whole system an MOT, and by taking these supplements and following a sugar-, gluten- and dairy-free diet I felt I was able to do this.

I've always been into exercise – before the wedding I worked out a lot because I wanted to look my best on our day – but now I began to do more gentle forms that help the mind as well as the body. It was important for me to keep calm and therefore I didn't want to put any burden on my adrenal glands with excessive exercise. Yoga, swimming and walking all allowed me to relax, which really helped to improve my mood, and because they were all things I enjoyed anyway, I made time to do them more often. In the beginning, I had to force myself to an extent, but very soon they became such a huge part of my day, something I looked forward to. Again, it wasn't about losing weight, but, bit by bit, I began to feel good about myself again, and even about the situation I was in.

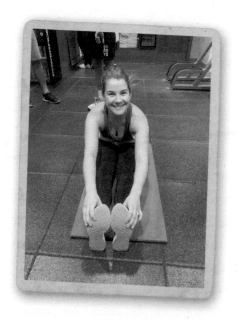

Part of my reboot involved taking gentle exercise.

I also began to practise mindfulness. Shortly after the wedding, and because I still struggled with anxiety, I'd read a book called *Calming Your Anxious Mind* by Jeffrey Brantley and Jon Kabat-Zinn. The message of the book, of mindfulness generally, is to be present. To keep bringing yourself back to the present moment, to 'now', rather than allowing yourself to spiral off into the future or dwell in the past. I'm sure this seems a very simple concept to some people but it was something of a revelation to me. Maybe I'd been told to do this previously but the message hadn't clicked. Reading this book, though, I could suddenly understand and relate to the idea much more. I began to try it, just sitting quietly, allowing thoughts to come and go, and I found it worked. It didn't cure my anxiety – I don't suppose anything ever fully will – but it certainly helped me to feel better and get a handle on my mind and the way it can spin out of my control.

During the six-month detox I got into the habit of meditating every morning. I'd get up and spend some time before breakfast breathing and quietening my mind. I've always been someone who gets up as soon as they wake up. I don't hit 'snooze' or struggle to get out of bed, and often wake to the feeling of adrenaline running through me, my heart and mind racing. Just by breathing consciously, I've discovered I can reset this, taking time to calm down and focus before the day runs away with me.

On warmer days, I'd go outside to the garden to practise; if it was too cold, I'd use the bedroom. In the beginning, I could only manage five minutes at a time because my mind whizzed so much, but gradually I improved and increased my concentration span until I was able to do twenty minutes without even noticing the time go by. I even went on a one-day meditation course and downloaded an app to my phone, Headspace, that provides guided meditations and mindfulness training.

I soon found I could tap into the feeling of peace more easily at other times of the day when I needed to. If I was confronted with a fearful situation, it became easier to get to a place where I could stop my mind from racing and just focus on my breath. And really, it's amazing how getting up and just breathing for a few minutes, before you do anything else with your day, changes the way you feel and respond to demanding situations. There's something quite spiritual about being able to connect to the world around you like that, and bring yourself to a state of calm.

Meditation isn't for everybody; that's not how everyone's mind works. Different things work for different people, whether it's going to the gym, running, just being outside – the important thing is to find something that works for you, and to stick with it. Like most things, I discovered that it takes practice!

Once I was meditating, exercising and eating well, I felt that my mind and body were mending, but I wanted to think about my spirit, too, and connecting to myself on a deeper level. I knew that was an important dimension to what I was doing, and I began to look around for inspiration, new ideas that attracted me and appealed to me, ways of thinking about my situation from another perspective. I've always liked quotes and sayings, combinations of words that offer a different point of view and feel as if they have the power to change your way of thinking. I wanted to find things that helped my mental outlook, that meant something to me.

During the one-day meditation course I went on, the teacher put a lot of emphasis on starting the day with a positive quote or an affirmation. That practice really appealed to me because I was beginning to understand just how much you can actually alter a situation simply by changing the way you think about it; that there is no such thing as 'reality', only the way we choose to see it. That was very comforting, reassuring and positive for me.

I found the idea that I didn't have to accept something as it initially appeared to me – that I could make it whatever I needed it to be – to be very empowering. I didn't have to feel helpless, or like a failure. I could look at my life, and myself, differently. As a result, I began to feel that I could reach acceptance of the situation I was in – emotionally and physically – rather than constantly fighting it, rejecting it, and wishing it was something different.

The funny thing was, as soon as I was open to the idea of finding messages that spoke to me and sparked my imagination, there they were: in shops, on Instagram, all around me. Some of the ones that helped me the most can be found on the inside covers of this book, in the hope that you might take something away from them too.

One of the first that I discovered was on a card that read 'amazing things will happen'. I think it came with something I'd ordered online. I opened the box and it tumbled out of the packaging. It was such a simple statement, and it was everything I now believed. As I'd started to feel better in myself, I'd begun to believe truly that I'd get pregnant some day, I just had to be patient. If it didn't happen immediately, that was OK because it *was* going to happen.

I felt that everything was leading towards a happy outcome, and that it would take as long as it took; I just had to keep trying and believing. Harry and I had always said to each other, 'We won't give up. We'll keep going, together, until we get there.'

Another affirmation I felt strongly about was one that read 'today is your day', which I found on a postcard and really identified with. Saying it made me believe that it could be my day because some day, it *would* be my turn.

I no longer looked with envy and bitterness at pregnant women and women with small babies. Instead, I actively wished something good for those women I saw. I'd think, 'I hope you have a healthy pregnancy and I hope your baby is safe' rather than 'Why is that not me?' And in doing so, I felt a thousand times better! The resentful feelings left me and I understood that we all have different paths in life. I realized that I didn't know what path had brought those women to this point, how hard it might have been for them. Now don't get me wrong, I still had my moments and it was tough, but I worked really hard to change my thoughts, and the affirmations helped enormously.

I'd started visiting an acupuncturist after our wedding but before we started trying for a baby, because I'd heard many times that acupuncture could do good things for both fertility and anxiety. I initially went for traditional acupuncture treatments, which I found relaxing and helpful, but then I heard from a friend about a guy called Gerad Kite, who I discovered had an amazing reputation in helping with fertility issues. He practises Five Element Acupuncture, whereby a patient's health is looked at not only as a whole but also through the lens of five elements: Water, Wood, Fire, Earth and Metal. Determining the weakest element in each patient is crucial for diagnosis. In other styles of acupuncture the needle is placed and left in an acupuncture point to sedate or calm for around 20 minutes. In five element acupuncture the needle is inserted to the depth of the acupuncture point and immediately removed.

I looked Gerad up online and found he'd also written a book called *The Art of Baby-Making*, which I read and really enjoyed while I was on holiday the summer after the wedding. It was interesting, very informative and left me feeling positive.

So during this time of detox I decided to book an appointment with Gerad and found him to be both spiritual and incredibly practical. He's treated so many women who haven't been able to get pregnant – often because of an underlying cause such as stress or trauma – and many times these women have fallen pregnant naturally following treatment by him. That wasn't my story, of course, but I did find the sessions with him extremely powerful. I'd feel a surge of energy during the treatment, as if things inside me were being unblocked, and would leave his clinic feeling on top of the world, or wonderfully calm, depending on what my body needed.

I went to see Gerad every six weeks or so during my six-month time-out (and also continued to see him during the IVF treatment and my pregnancy with Lola). Acupuncture was a therapy I chose to invest in during that time, and Gerad is someone I feel everyone should see once in their life. My wellbeing improved hugely whenever I'd been to visit him and he was also somebody I could talk to. He was a wonderful and important piece of the puzzle.

As part of my detox, I also asked myself the question, what is going to make me happy? The answer was, as it always has been, music. I'd left Escala before getting married because I was planning on having a family, but also because I felt I'd done as much with that career as I wanted to, and was ready to move on. I'd achieved more than I'd ever expected to and knew I'd always be able to look back and be proud of that time. But I was ready for something different.

It would've been very difficult to go back to being a professional classical musician after my time with Escala. I hadn't played classical violin for ten years – with Escala we performed on electric instruments and our repertoire was all crossover – so I didn't feel anywhere near the standard I would have needed to be, and it would've taken a lot of hard work to return to that calibre.

Also, it's very difficult to get back into the world of professional classical music once you've left it. It's highly competitive, with only so many opportunities to go round, and fundamentally it wasn't what I wanted. Harry's career was unpredictable and involved a lot of time away on tour – if we'd both been living that kind of life, we'd barely have seen each other, or been able to plan anything at all. In fact, I wanted to do something completely different and keep music as a hobby. So I joined amateur orchestras and was able to play my violin again, which I loved. My dad also played in these orchestras, and it was a real pleasure to be able to share that time with him.

The effect of changing my diet, of exercising more but gently, and of meditating and repeating positive affirmations was wonderful. It completely changed the way I felt, both mentally and physically. I went from being unhappy and in despair, to feeling bright and energetic. But there was one more thing I needed to do, and in a funny way it was the hardest thing, because it wasn't a question of will-power, it was a matter of changing something fundamental about myself.

I realized that, for a short time, I was going to have to reverse my natural instinct to put everyone else first and myself last. I was going to have to be 'selfish', even though I firmly believe that's the wrong word because it sounds so negative. I was going to have to prioritize myself for a change, and save my energy for me and the baby I so badly wanted.

It wasn't easy. I've always wanted to give – it's what I've done all my life. My mum is an incredibly generous, warm person, who has always thought about others far more than herself, and I'd seen her do that for as long as I could remember; it was my normal. I was determined, though, that this time off was for me, and was what I needed to do in

A whole new me

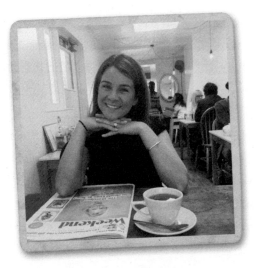

Time to put myself first!

order to have a baby. Instead of running around after other people, falling in with their plans, doing things for them, I needed to step back. I needed to learn to say 'no'.

Of course when you're not working – and by then I'd closed my online gift shop, Izzy's Attic – everyone thinks you have all the time in the world. People can take advantage, even when they don't mean to. Often, I wasn't even able to give a reason for not meeting someone, or helping with something, because only our families and closest friends knew what we'd been going through. I just had to tell people I was having a busy month, which most of my friends were fine with, but it must have seemed a little odd that I was never around as I'm usually the person who always says yes. I suppose real friends just know that there's something happening in your life, even if you haven't specifically told them what. They instinctively understand and leave you be, they don't pressure you.

Saying no to people was liberating and refreshing, and when my six months drew to a close, I began to fully reap the rewards of the changes I'd made and the time off I'd given myself. I was now at a point where I knew I was ready to move forward.

Despite feeling so well, my periods hadn't come back – they'd stopped again as soon as I finished taking the Clomid. So I still had no menstrual cycle to speak of, and therefore, in my mind, it felt that conceiving naturally wasn't going to happen any time soon. After a great deal of thought I told Harry that I wanted to have IVF.

I knew that it was something I wanted to try – and sooner rather than later. Initially, Harry wasn't keen. He thought I was leaping ahead too much, that we didn't need to go that far, that we should wait a little longer. He'd always been more inclined to see how things played out because, as he said, 'We're both young, there's no rush.' He was right, but I wasn't willing to give it any longer.

He listened to me as I explained why I didn't want to wait. Didn't dare to wait. Nothing was happening and I didn't believe I had any chance of falling pregnant naturally. Also, I wasn't just thinking about having one baby, I was thinking about a family.

I suppose Harry was nervous that I might revert to the panicked state I'd got myself into during the first year of trying for a baby. He didn't want me to undo all the hard work I'd put in to feeling calmer. As usual, he was trying to be rational for both of us. I reassured him that my frame of mind was different now – I was keen to move on to this next stage, but with more understanding and patience. I was mentally and physically prepared.

As a cautious first step, in September 2014 we went to see my gynaecologist for a chat about what IVF would entail. Harry and I both agreed that we wouldn't commit to anything there and then, but would take the following month to think things over carefully.

I still remember the day we decided, together, that we would go ahead with IVF. It was just over a month later, in November, and having made our decision, Harry and I went for a beautiful walk in Richmond Park. As we walked, I looked up to see the sun shining through the clouds and I felt so full of hope. Harry took a photo of me, and when I

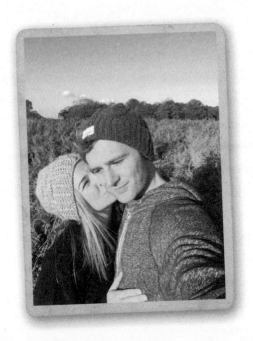

The day Harry and I decided to go ahead with IVF.

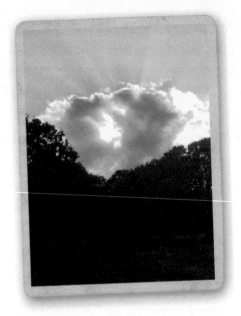

*I hoped the stork-shaped cloud
was a positive sign for us.*

saw it, I realized that the clouds behind my head had formed the shape of a stork. I knew in that moment that we were making the right decision. I felt as if the universe had spoken to me.

I kept that photo with me throughout our IVF treatment and had it with me when I injected myself with the fertility drugs. I even took it into the clinic. That photo, for me, signified hope.

9

IVF

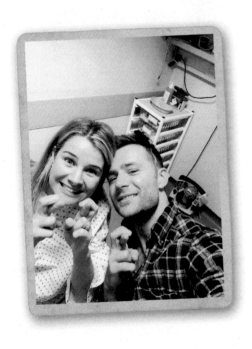

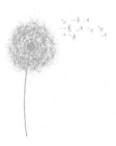

FOR ALL THAT I believed, and still believe, that the stork-shaped cloud Harry and I saw was a sign, and for all the certainty I had that this was what I wanted, IVF still felt like something huge and terrifying.

It actually stands for 'in vitro fertilization', meaning the medical procedure whereby an egg is fertilized by sperm in a lab dish. But what it meant to me, personally, was that Harry and I had accepted we wouldn't conceive naturally nor with minimal interventions – drug stimulation, fallopian-tube flushing or IUI. We were, therefore, moving on to our remaining option.

Because of this, IVF could have felt like a last chance. Instead, I was determined to stay in the optimistic mindset I'd worked so hard to reach, and to view it differently. So I made the decision that we wouldn't treat it as if we were approaching the end of the road, but feel instead that we had made a choice, and that we had a real chance. I deliberately went into IVF thinking how positive a time it would be – how wonderful that we had an opportunity to do something, to take action, to change the outcome of our future. It was the start of a new journey with the prospect of hope at the end, hope that I would fall pregnant and we would have our longed-for baby.

I strongly believe that, despite the general lack of knowledge and understanding surrounding IVF, it shouldn't be looked on as something frightening, invasive or intrusive; a horrible obstacle to clear before the joy of having a baby. IVF, I've always thought, is an amazing gift and I'm very grateful that it was an option for us. I've thought so many times of the women in the days before it was available as a treatment, who couldn't have children naturally and had no other options, and the effect that had on their lives.

Once we decided that we were going ahead with IVF, I felt so much relief. After wondering and considering for a long time, it was a decision I was happy with. We told both our families, I told my best friend, Chantal, and Harry told a couple of his closest friends. Other friends vaguely knew there was something going on, but we chose not to be fully open with them. To some extent, I changed my mind about this later on, when time and circumstances showed me a different perspective and I came to believe that more openness was better, but during the first round of IVF, Harry and I both preferred to keep the circle of people who knew very small.

IVF

We made that choice partly because we didn't know exactly what the treatment would involve – what the medical process would be – so to think about explaining to others what we didn't understand fully ourselves was hard to contemplate. But also, I just wanted to be in my own bubble and focus on what I needed to do. I felt very much that this was my time and whether the outcome I longed for happened on the first attempt, or five attempts down the line, I knew I needed to concentrate and do everything in my power to give it the best possible shot. All my energy needed to go into this; there would be nothing left over. I knew that family and our closest friends would understand that.

The ability to put myself first, which I'd learned during the six months of detox, was something that I chose to continue when we went into IVF, because I knew I needed to. I gave myself permission to be selfish again. I do think that most of us need an excuse to do that. These days, when I talk to other women who are about to begin IVF, this is one of the first things I suggest: take time to consider what is important to you and what you need to do in order to get through the process as best you can. Take the time to do things that will make you happy rather than things to keep others happy.

For me, the hardest part of our decision was finally accepting that I needed help to get pregnant; that my body wasn't going to do it alone. I found that difficult, certainly at first, because of the way it made me feel – like a failure, not properly a woman. But I gradually changed the way I thought about this and altered my viewpoint to become more philosophical: this is what I want and this is what I have to do to get it. I believed that, with help, I would get pregnant. From the very beginning, my gynaecologist had said that my issues were treatable. Of course no doctor can guarantee you a baby, but mine always said there was hope. Plenty of hope.

So I chose to see IVF as something helpful, and tried to focus only on all the good things. Of course it's frightening too and the reality is that the medical profession can only take you so far. They can stimulate egg production, harvest the eggs, choose the best possible, and fertilize them with the best possible sperm – all of which is amazing – but the minute a fertilized egg is put back into your body, then all over again it's your body that is responsible for carrying on the job. And there's always the possibility that your body won't do the next bit. For this reason, I forced myself not to leap too far ahead and think of the negative possibilities, but instead to take things step by step.

The first decision we faced was which fertility clinic we would go to. Harry and I felt so incredibly fortunate that at this time in our lives we were in a position to have treatment privately. I understand that this isn't everyone's experience.

My gynaecologist had a couple of fertility clinics that he was linked to, but was happy for us to find and choose one we both felt most comfortable with. We did do a little research around statistics and outcomes for the different places, but there is so much behind the numbers – including patients' age, the cause of their infertility as well as how many people have used the clinic – that it wasn't the route we ultimately took. I wanted to be treated somewhere I felt safe, happy and relaxed. I needed a personal connection with my doctors in order to feel that way. We considered several options and in the end went for a clinic called Herts & Essex Fertility Centre, just outside London. It felt right and we were both comforted to know Dr Ram was a consultant there. Also, with Harry being in the public eye, we both felt better being treated away from the city; somewhere a bit quieter and more discreet.

At first I felt a bit embarrassed to be going to a fertility clinic at my age. I'd always thought that it was women in their forties who went for IVF because of age-related issues – how totally naive of me. I worried the clinic would think I was very young to be having treatment, but of course there was no judgement from anyone there. There are so many reasons why couples might need to have IVF but I never knew this until my own fertility journey began.

One of the clinic's kind nurses came to my gynaecologist's office in London and talked us right through the process, explaining everything that would happen to me, and why. She was very compassionate and explained it all to us fully and calmly. Even so, I went home that night and the first thing I did was write everything down, so I understood what was about to happen. There was so much information to take in, I found it overwhelming. Being somebody who loves to be organized, having it on paper in black and white helped me to feel prepared, and I therefore felt more relaxed about it.

The staff at fertility clinics are living IVF day in day out, but for me it was like learning a new language. I went over and over my dates for the various stages, and looked up every medication I was being prescribed so that I knew with one hundred per cent certainty what I was about to put in my body. Each clinic has a different protocol, so even though Google did help a little, it also confused me. But Herts & Essex answered any questions I had and never made me feel silly for asking.

The first thing that has to happen during the long protocol, which is what I was put on, is that you need to have a period. You're usually asked to take the contraceptive pill for twenty-one days to bring it on. Which is a strange thing in itself – just when you want to get started, to get pregnant you have to go back on the Pill! The logic behind it is to 'reset' your menstrual cycle to allow the doctors to control the timing of the IVF cycle, because from then on, in my case, every hormone needed throughout the process would be synthetic and self-administered. It also decreases the chances of cysts forming in the ovaries, which is a particular risk for women with PCOS.

I'd actually started taking the Pill a month beforehand, while we were still making our final decision. This meant we were able to move on to the next stage of the cycle without delay once we decided to go ahead. (If we'd chosen not to, then there was always the chance it might have prompted the return of my periods, which hadn't come back during my detox.)

At the same time as taking the Pill, I wanted to carry on with what I saw as my job in all of this – to take charge of anything I could so as to be in the best shape possible,

IVF

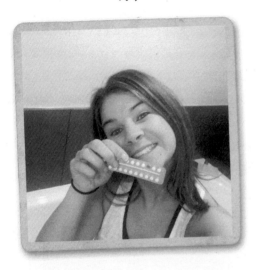

*It's always a big moment when you start
your medication for IVF.*

mentally and physically, to support the medical process.
The drugs I was about to take were hardcore, and the
process can be draining, so I used those twenty-one days
to find out everything I could about what would help to
support me holistically.

I left nothing to chance. I was willing to try anything I
thought would give me the best possible chance of having a
successful round of IVF, and which would keep me calm and
happy within myself. I'd already discovered that changing
my diet, exercising in a certain way and meditating had
had a profound effect on me. I wanted to go further and
learn more.

More than anything, I wanted to feel that I wasn't passive
in all of this, a body to be injected and controlled. I wanted
my role in making this dream come true to be an active

one. In some ways, I approached IVF in the same way I'd approached learning the violin – if I wanted to get the best result I possibly could, I had to prepare. And I really believe that all the things I did helped – maybe they didn't have much to do with getting the result I wanted (although in my own mind I believe they did), but they certainly helped me cope with the process.

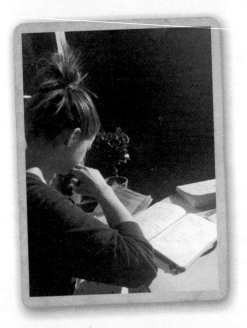

Throughout my treatment, I researched extensively
so that I was fully prepared.

I continued to take specific vitamins and minerals to help with the quality of my eggs. I got my hands on a brilliant fertility nutrition book, which gave me a detailed plan of exactly what to eat at each stage of the cycle. For example, during the stimulation phase, which is when you're injecting hormones to encourage the growth of the follicles in your ovaries, it's also a good idea to eat lots of blood-nourishing food to help thicken the lining of the womb, so that when they put the fertilized egg back, the lining is as receptive as possible. There's a number of such books out there, but the one I read was *Fertile* by Emma Cannon, a fertility, pregnancy and women's health expert. (I've included more details of my diet and other alternative supports on page 259.)

One of my quirkier ideas, according to Harry, was something called oil pulling. This involved putting a spoonful of coconut oil into my mouth each morning, then swilling it around for ten minutes before spitting it out, to cleanse the mouth of bacteria and toxins. He'd tease me about it and on one occasion I had to spit the oil out fast because we got the giggles so badly!

A much more conventional change was making sure that I slept as much as I needed, and avoided stressful and emotional situations as much as possible. I also carried on with my mindfulness practice. Every day I'd mentally do a full body scan, turning my attention to all the different parts of my body and relaxing each one in turn. Sometimes – I admit it! – I'd have a little doze while doing it, but even so, the simple act of breathing properly deeply centred me, and was a huge lifeline in dealing with any anxious thoughts. I also listened to guided meditation sessions by Zita West, a fertility specialist who has a clinic in London and whose holistic approach to fertility treatment I like, as well as one by Maggie Howell called *The IVF Companion*. I'd often fall asleep at night to the comforting sound of her voice.

Zita West's guided meditations talk you through exactly what happens during each stage of an IVF cycle, which I found very helpful. I like to understand and be able to imagine what's happening inside my body, and she's very good at giving a verbal picture of what's taking place during all the different phases, which makes it much easier to connect with it all. There's a long patch in the middle of the meditation where it's quiet, and during that time I'd repeat positive affirmations and visualize my body accepting our embryo as if in a warm hug, arms stretched out, and welcoming it to its new home.

I carried on reading and reciting affirmations, even outside of the meditations, and would keep reminders of them at strategic spots around the house. I'd catch sight of them and remember to stay in a good place mentally and not let my mind spiral towards too many 'what ifs' or negative thoughts. The hardest part of IVF for me was the not knowing and uncertainty around the outcome, and because of this, remaining positive was my biggest challenge.

At this time, as part of the gentle exercise I'd do, I'd go for lots of walks. I've always enjoyed being around nature and things that grow, and I found it helpful to be outside. One of my daily walks would be around a square near where we lived. It will always remain a magical place for me, a space where I was able to find peace and quiet in my busy mind, and to think positively.

A robin used to appear while I walked, day after day, and follow me about. I read somewhere about a legend that says they're inhabited by the souls of people who've passed away but come and visit us. For me, that little robin was my granny; I felt her presence, which I very much needed just then.

I dearly loved that time. In many ways, I don't think I'd ever been so well as I was during the months of my detox and preparing for my IVF cycle. I'd spent so many years being miserable, on edge, fearful for the future, agitated because I wanted a baby so much and it wasn't happening, and feeling bad about myself. I shut all that down, reconnected with myself, and prepared my body for what I believed would follow. I felt as if I was being proactive, and making decisions that I hoped would bring great results.

Going through an IVF cycle you learn there are many stages, especially being on the long protocol as I was. There are many different bridges to cross, different things to do as the days and weeks go on. This means that, instead of thinking only about the end result, your mind is focused on the short term – 'Today I've got to do this. Tomorrow we've got to get to that scan' – so living day by day helped me to stay present and in the moment. If my mind drifted into the future (as it likes to do), I tried my best to bring it back to the moment and focus.

I'd spent so long not being present, passing all the imaginary milestones I'd set for myself – 'Will I be pregnant for that wedding? My birthday? Christmas? Next summer?' – and the answer always being, 'No. No. No. No.' Disappointment after disappointment. Now, I was learning to keep my mind in check and stop myself from looking too far into the future.

After almost a month of taking the Pill, I had a procedure

done called endometrial pipelle sampling. This is when the doctor inserts a thin tube through the cervix and deliberately scratches the lining of the womb. This is done because there's evidence that it stimulates the lining to be more receptive to accepting an embryo. It also gave Dr Ram a chance to draw a diagram of my awkward-shaped cervix and backward-tilting womb, which was then helpful to him during egg collection.

At this point I was given a drug called Suprecur, which shut down production of my normal follicle-stimulating hormones (it basically puts you into early menopause) before I started the stimulation phase. Once my ovaries were quiet and ready for stimulation, the Gonal-F injections began.

I was put on a high dose of the drug to stimulate egg production and initially the clinic was worried about over-stimulation. Having PCOS increases your risk of this happening so there were concerns. It can cause a serious condition called Ovarian Hyperstimulation Syndrome (OHSS), which means your ovaries overreact to the drugs and produce too many follicles. Therefore, at the first sign of it happening, the doctors will cancel the IVF cycle. However, because I'd already had an IUI (when I was given a lower dose of Gonal-F) that had failed, my gynaecologist insisted that I needed a higher dose in order for my ovaries to respond.

The injecting isn't pleasant but it wasn't as bad as I had anticipated – one evening I had to do it in the loos at one of Harry's gigs – and luckily I'm not afraid of needles. However, it does get sore, and you do have to keep going back to the same spots. Gonal-F and Suprecur are both injected into the stomach, so it's hard to find new places in that one small area. As I responded badly to Clomid I was worried how I would react to the IVF drugs. I did suffer badly with bloating, but in general I felt well, which I was very grateful for. All this time I kept my stork photo and the 'amazing things will happen' card with me, and as I injected the drugs I would think to myself, 'Thank you. Amazing things *will* happen.'

I was also prescribed 75mg of aspirin daily. It's believed that aspirin helps to keep the blood thin and prevents it from clotting. This not only helps blood flow to the lining of the womb to help endometrial thickness and therefore implantation, but it also supports a pregnancy.

Throughout this period of the process, which takes around two weeks, you go for regular scans where they check your ovaries and womb lining. I always felt nervous beforehand, praying that my body was responding well. And each time I went, luckily everything was progressing as it should – in part thanks to the massive beetroot risottos I was eating, I'm sure, because beetroot is very blood nourishing and helps the lining of the womb to thicken! Seeing the scans and knowing that the drugs were working helped me to feel positive and confident, and each time I left the clinic, I reminded myself to take one step at a time.

While I was happy with my progress, I was still incredibly nervous about a part of the process still to come – egg collection – which has to happen under heavy sedation. It's not a full general anaesthetic but you're still out cold. For someone with anxiety, the idea of being unconscious is terrifying. You're obviously completely lacking control, in an unfamiliar environment, with your legs in the air – and the area under fire is your most private place. By this time I was very used to being checked and examined, but the prospect of this procedure felt very different because I'd be unconscious throughout; I was horribly frightened that I wouldn't wake up.

I was also worried about the fact that you can't eat before you're sedated. If I don't eat for a while I can get shaky, leading to an adrenaline spike, which in turn can bring on my anxiety. I practised mindfulness and did positive visualizations to help with the way I felt, but ultimately it was going to be my biggest challenge to overcome.

About thirty-six hours before egg collection, once we knew the eggs were reaching their optimum size, I was given something called a hCG trigger shot – essentially a dose of human chorionic gonadotrophin – to help mature the eggs and get them ready for retrieval.

I explained to the team at the clinic how I felt about being sedated, and they were kind enough to schedule my egg collection as early in the day as they could, and gave me so much reassurance. One of the nurses, Sarah, told me that she would be with me throughout the procedure. The last thing I said to her before going under was, 'Will you hold my hand?' She did, and I'll be eternally grateful to her. She was wonderful.

Harry was by my side, as always, but this time he had a job to do too – fill a phial with sperm. This was the big day for his part of the deal as well! Which I'm sure isn't nice, but let's not forget it was the only thing he had to do, physically speaking, and he was able to do it in private.

After egg collection, I was wheeled back to my cubicle, and I came round very quickly. Too quickly, really. I was in a lot of discomfort – it feels like a really bad period pain, deep inside you. I was also in floods of tears. As I regained consciousness, I kept saying, 'I feel so sorry for Rupert!' Of course the nurse didn't know what I was talking about, and Harry wasn't there at that point to explain or comfort me. I've heard since that coming round from being sedated can spark very strong emotional reactions. While I don't remember being in control of my tears or my thoughts, I know I've never felt emotion like that.

Amazingly, they collected twenty-one eggs, which was a high number and verging on over-stimulation. Luckily, it was OK and we were able to go ahead with the rest of the cycle.

We then had to wait until the next day to hear how our eggs were doing and whether they had fertilized. The insemination process the clinic used with us is something called ICSI – intracytoplasmic sperm injection. This means that instead of simply putting the eggs and sperm together in a dish and allowing a sperm to find its way to each egg and fertilize it 'naturally', each mature egg is held with a specialized pipette and a very delicate, sharp, hollow needle is used to pick up a single sperm. The needle with the sperm is then carefully inserted through the shell of the egg and into the cytoplasm before the sperm is released. The point of doing this is to enhance the chances of success.

Thirteen of our twenty-one eggs were fertilized successfully and were now referred to as zygotes (although to me they were our embies!). The day of fertilization is referred to as Day Zero and the following day, Day One, we had twelve zygotes because one did not survive. Up until Day Three, the clinic rang every day between 8.30 and 9 a.m. and told us how our eggs were doing. We made great friends with the embryologists and put a lot of trust in them as they were taking care of our most fragile possessions.

Between Days Four and Five, the zygote becomes a blastocyst, which means it becomes a far more complex structure of approximately 200 cells. In a 'natural' pregnancy, the blastocyst phase is the development stage just before implantation in the lining of the mother's uterus, and it can be delicate. Some zygotes don't survive the transition to blastocyst. Because of this, if I'd had only a few fertilized eggs, my doctors may have recommended transferring one on Day Three, but because I had twelve they felt they could justify the risk of waiting until Day Five before transferring.

The clinic doesn't look at the embryos on Day Four as it's difficult to distinguish a degenerating embryo from one which is progressing towards a blastocyst. So on Day Four, when we didn't get a phone call, it felt suddenly strange. The day felt horribly long but then, on Day Five, we got the all-important news: three blastocysts had survived out of twelve. After all that time, with twenty-one eggs collected and thirteen fertilized, we had three viable blastocysts. Sometimes, when I think about how hard it is to conceive,

I wonder that anyone manages it naturally! I remember feeling completely overwhelmed that day, and so incredibly lucky to be going into the next stage with three blastocysts. Again, I was very conscious about taking each day as it came but it felt as if I'd cleared one of the higher hurdles.

During the five-day wait, I was put on a drug called Cyclogest, a form of progesterone, which your body needs in order to encourage a pregnancy to progress. It's when your progesterone level drops that you have a period. When you're pregnant, though, it keeps rising, so taking the drug mimics carefully what would naturally happen in your body.

Initially, I was given the Cyclogest in pessary form, and I reacted really badly to it. I was bloated to the point where I couldn't stand. I was so uncomfortable that I had to lie in bed – if I stood up I was bent over double – in misery, with very painful stomach cramps because progesterone slows down your digestive system too. It felt as if someone was twisting my stomach. I stuck with it for a few days but it didn't get any better, so I switched to a different brand of progesterone called Crinone. I responded much better but even so, on transfer day, which is when the blastocyst is placed back into the womb, I still felt very uncomfortable – bloated and sore.

We went back to the clinic on Day Five, after receiving the exciting phone call giving the go-ahead for transfer, and the remaining two blastocysts were frozen the following day, Day Six. Psychologically, it was comforting to know that we had three chances of a successful pregnancy, with two waiting patiently in the freezer if this first one didn't succeed.

Dare to dream

Harry was supposed to be on *This Morning* that day, but of course he came with me instead. We were so excited – it was the first time during all the fertility treatments that there was some certainty. We weren't turning up to a scan to see whether I had responded to the drugs or not. We'd made it to this stage and it felt incredible. There was a fertilized egg waiting, ready to go back home where it belonged, safe and sound. I had so longed for this moment and believed that, even if this round failed and our little embryo only stayed there a few days, it would still be a miracle to have had life inside me for that time.

Before the embryo is transferred, the remains of the progesterone gel has to be cleaned away, so there's a bit of swabbing and mopping to be done, which isn't very pleasant. By then, though, all my dignity had pretty much been stripped away and my most private area had been examined so often that it had become as impersonal as a hand or a foot. I got changed into my gown, and Harry and I went into a very sterile white room, which has an ultrasound monitor so that you can see exactly what's happening during the transfer. It's all very clinical – a hatch opens between the lab and the treatment room, and the dish with your embryo in it is checked with the doctor to verify your names, then you're told that you'll see your embryo on the screen, projected from the microscope – but to us, it was the closest to magic we've ever been. It wasn't the romantic way you assume it will be when you conceive for the first time, but for us it was every bit as romantic. It was life, new life, happening right in front of us.

IVF

To see our embryo on the screen was just mind blowing, for me and for Harry. It looked like a beautiful full moon that had been magnified and we could see the craters. We were so moved. This was our baby. The embryo is tiny, a speck, not even the size of a sesame seed, and they transfer it using a long thin catheter. We watched as the catheter went in, and as the doctor released it there was a flash of light on the monitor. I remember thinking it looked like a shooting star. 'That's it!' he said. As soon as the embryo is released and the catheter withdrawn, it's done. At this point the embryologist checks under the microscope that the embryo hasn't been retained in the catheter.

Immediately, you can stand up, walk around, go to the loo, but I didn't want to move off the bed – somehow I thought by lying there it would give our little embryo a

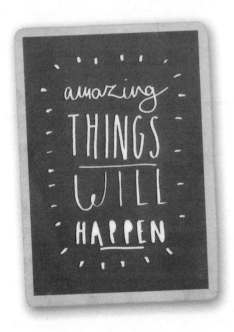

better chance. Of course this isn't the case and it's very safe to move. The only thing you're not advised to do is to lift anything heavy, which for me, in my head, meant lifting nothing – Harry even carried my handbag out of the clinic that day!

Harry and I were totally amazed – we hadn't expected to feel so overwhelmed with emotion. It was a moment we'll never forget, and it was beautiful to share the magic together – the world stopped for a second. For us it felt as if this little life was home, at last.

10

An agonizing wait

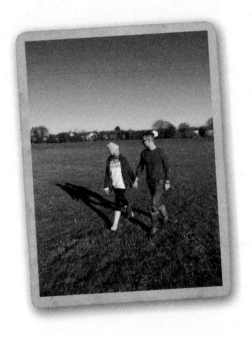

COMING HOME from the clinic after the embryo transfer was wonderful; knowing I finally had life inside me. As soon as I was through the front door, I said to Harry, 'I really want a bacon sandwich!' After all the beetroot risottos, the healthy smoothies and long walks, suddenly all I felt like was a bacon sandwich and bed.

I'd been told not to do a pregnancy test for two weeks, and that wait – to see whether the embryo had successfully implanted, whether I was actually pregnant – was very challenging. I had an amazing sense of warmth all over, but also wondered how I would get through the coming fortnight. Two weeks of waiting, wondering whether the embryo would make itself at home and whether my body would keep hold of it, trying to stay positive and not leap ahead mentally. I didn't know how I would manage,

I just knew that I had to. Up until then, something had been happening nearly every day. The clinic were in touch constantly, I was having scans, assessments and injections. I'd been busy, proactive, on a mission, and suddenly there we were, left alone, with nothing to do but wait.

I'd been told the date I could do the pregnancy test – 10 December – and I just had to be patient until then. Everything had gone as well as it could have up to that point. The transferred embryo was grade B, which was good, the lining of my womb was nice and thick, and I was a good candidate statistically in terms of my age and general health. There was every reason to believe this would work.

I was so in tune with my body by this stage that every cramp, every twinge, every backache, every headache, resonated. Just to confuse things, as I was still taking the progesterone, everything I felt was indeed like a pregnancy symptom.

I needed to stay calm, and so I knew that this was the time to continue what I'd been doing – the mindfulness, the meditation, the walking and immersing myself in nature. I tapped into very gentle yoga – breathing and stretching, really. I listened to hypno-visualizations, which I found very relaxing. I would envisage the embryo implanting by creating an image in my mind – I would see the roots of a tree coming out of the lining of my womb, ready to embrace it, and I would tell it, 'I'm going to hold you, you're safe, I have you.' That helped me by keeping my mind calm, and by giving me something to do that I believed was helpful.

Really though, for all the distractions I tried, I was just counting down the days. Harry would ask me how I was and I'd say I was fine, but I think we each knew how the other was really feeling. It was hard for him, too, just having to wait, with nothing that he could usefully do, particularly given that he's a person who likes to be proactive. And so we kept each other company – lots of cosy nights in, just the two of us, watching films and listening to music. It was coming up to Christmas, which is a time of year I've always loved, so I finished the Christmas shopping, listened to carols and wrapped presents. I decorated the tree and the house. I embraced it all.

For ages I'd wanted to put together an album of photos and memories from our wedding, and finally this time seemed the perfect opportunity to do that. It was also just the right time, sitting by the fire one afternoon, to look through all the messages our wedding guests had written and

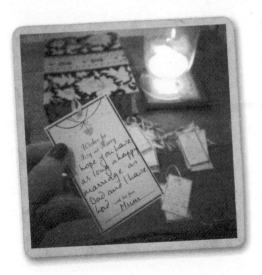

My mum's wish from the wishing tree
at our wedding.

hung on the wishing tree. It was such a happy experience to be able to read the kind and beautiful things that people we love had written and hoped for us. My mum's wish was 'I hope you have as long and happy a marriage as Dad and I have had', and this made my heart smile.

It was also the time of year when everyone is waiting to see the John Lewis Christmas advert for the first time. Harry and I always watch it together – it's a little tradition of ours. This was the year of Monty the Penguin, and oh, how I cried, wondering all the while if my response was a pregnancy symptom.

I have two Ragdoll cats called Murphy and Morris. Both are full of personality (and don't always enjoy each other's company!) but Murphy has a particular sort of intuition. I've found, in the ten years I've had him, that he's often nearby when I need him to be. During those two weeks he stuck to me like glue. Wherever I was in the house, there he was, beside me, as close as he could get.

It's a funny thing, who you feel you can talk to when you go through IVF. Everybody's different, of course, but I found it very difficult to open up to anybody about it. My mum knew – I've always told her everything. She's my best friend and I don't think I could hide anything from her, but sometimes I worried about how all of this made her feel. I knew how hard it was for her too and I didn't want to cause her any upset. She felt everything for me almost as much as I felt it for myself.

I managed to talk to my best friend, Chantal, who was,

of course, a tower of strength. Chunny was four months pregnant at the time, and I longed for us to be pregnant together, but I tried not to put pressure on myself, even though it was hard not to run away with dreams that our children would grow up together and be best friends, just like us! Chunny was always very sensitive when it came to how much she talked about her pregnancy, and waited for me to ask any questions – of course I asked loads! There were moments that I found difficult, and at those times, even though Chunny was going through this wonderful period in her own life, I still felt she put my feelings first.

Harry's mum, Emma, was also a huge comfort and support to both of us. It must've been difficult for her to judge just how much to get involved and how many questions to ask – the relationship between a mother- and daughter-in-law

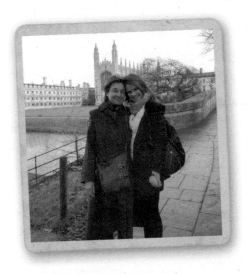

Harry's mum, Emma, was a huge support to us as we went through IVF.

is different to that between a mother and a daughter – but we're very close and open with each other. Emma's brother Mark died tragically in a car accident when he was twenty-seven, and she and I have always been able to talk honestly and share the grief about how that kind of tragedy affects a family; something that gave us a special bond very quickly. I feel so lucky to have such a loving and caring mother-in-law.

Another close family friend, who went through many traumatic years of IVF before finally having a baby, was also kind and helpful. It was she who first said to me that I needed to be selfish and put myself first. She encouraged me to ask her questions about the process, and she shared her experiences openly. I'm so thankful to her for being there for me. It was wonderful to have her to talk to, because you can't ask your doctors every single thing that occurs to you, and the internet can be a terrible thing – too much information with no way to process it properly.

Talking to even one person who's had IVF, who understands it and who understands you, is so important, and I hope everyone who reads this book has such a person in their lives. Of course, you deal with what you're going through in your own way, but a confidante with personal experience can be a huge help. In fact, one of the inspirations for writing this book was the number of people who got in touch, after Harry and I first opened up about our IVF experience, to say that they didn't have anyone they could share their own stories with. Hearing that made me want to normalize IVF, to talk about it openly and as something not to be ashamed of.

An agonizing wait

For anyone who reads this as a friend or family member of someone having IVF, or who they suspect is having difficulty conceiving, my advice is if you don't know what to say, have the honesty to admit it. It's OK to let someone know you're there, if they do want to talk, but don't try to rush in and 'fix' what they're going through. Sometimes people just need the space to talk – you don't need to feel as if you have to have a solution to their problem. For me, what I appreciated most was sensitivity and understanding.

Even though Harry and I had support, ultimately it was the love and warmth we felt from each other that was the best medicine for us both.

The two weeks passed somehow, and after what seemed like an eternity the day of the pregnancy test arrived. It needs to be done with the first wee of the morning, because that's when levels of the hCG hormone are at their highest concentration.

The night before, 9 December, my parents, Harry and I went to Cadogan Hall in London, where Rupert was playing a solo in a concert in aid of The Children's Trust, something he does every Christmas. It was a cold winter evening and Harry and I were both feeling incredibly nervous about the next day, so it was a great distraction to get out of the house and spend some time with family, listening to beautiful music. Being a charity event, it also helped to put things into perspective. We met many inspiring families there that evening. And of course, being in Rupert's company would cheer anyone up – he's my biggest reminder to appreciate what we have! An amazing piece of music was performed during the concert, 'Quanta Qualia' by Patrick Hawes, which I'd never heard before but loved. When I got home that evening I downloaded it immediately.

Before we left, Dad, who even though he's a man of few words always knows what to say at the right moment, said to me, 'You're glowing, Izzy!' I love that he said that. It must have been tough for him – he knew how nervous I felt and I'm sure both he and my mum felt the nerves for us too.

I'd been living for the moment of the test for far longer than the two weeks since the embryo transfer, but I refused to let myself think beyond doing it. It was still a question of going step by step – I couldn't begin to contemplate the many things that had to happen after that. I had to remind myself to cross each bridge as I came to it – I could only hope for the test to be positive.

Many women will say, 'I knew, I had a feeling', about being pregnant. Not me. I had no idea, no feeling, no gut instinct. I didn't know what was going to happen when I weed on that stick. I wasn't waiting to have a suspicion confirmed; I was waiting to be told either way.

After a few hours of broken sleep, I got up at about 5.30 a.m. and woke Harry. I couldn't stop my legs from shaking with nerves. I felt breathless and horribly anxious. Not one part of me was excited – I was far too nervous. I went into the bathroom clutching my cloud photo and my 'amazing things' card – I knew that I needed something positive with me in case the result wasn't what I longed for. I propped them both up on the sink, did the test and waited.

An agonizing wait

I could hardly breathe. My heart was thumping as I started to count down the three minutes. For the first time in my life, after countless pregnancy tests, I could see a second line coming through immediately. It was really, really faint but it was there. I was pregnant. I didn't cry, though – even then, I found it difficult to – but I was so excited, so totally overjoyed that I felt as if I was floating. I was on cloud nine.

Harry, from the beginning, was nervous. He didn't like that the line wasn't stronger, but I was happy and explained to him it was early days and that the line would get darker over the next few days. Running through my mind were the words 'We've done it!' There had been times when I didn't believe that I could – that my body could – but it had happened.

I called my parents, who had probably barely slept either, and told them the news. Then Harry rang his parents too, even though he didn't feel ready to celebrate properly. It wasn't that he knew something was wrong, but he would have liked more reassurance, and until he got it he wasn't fully able to let go and embrace the result.

Despite Harry's worries, it was a really joyful morning. He and I don't go out for dinner much, for us it's always about breakfast or brunch, so we put on our woolly hats and went to the coffee shop at the end of the road. They have an incentive where, once you've filled up your loyalty card with stamps, you get to spin a wheel and win a prize. That morning, we filled up our loyalty card. I was feeling lucky so I decided to spin the wheel and sure enough, I won the best prize possible – five free coffees.

When someone once asked me how I felt that day, the only way I could describe it was to say that for the first time I dared to dream. I had never ever dared to before then. I'd been holding myself back, always – too frightened, too aware of the possibilities of disappointment – but finally the day had come when I dared. When I could walk past the woman with the pram and smile at her, thinking, 'That'll be me.' When I could walk past the shops selling baby stuff and peer into their windows, believing that soon I would need it all. I no longer felt the pain of looking at things that weren't meant for me.

I rang my gynaecologist, who said he was delighted for us but rightly remained cautious. He said that he didn't need to see me yet, but that he wanted me to have a blood test to confirm the positive result and to book a scan for when I was seven weeks pregnant.

I did two more pregnancy tests that day because I needed reassurance that I would still see that second line appearing. Every few days from then on I would test to check the result was still positive. Of course I started looking out for signs and symptoms straight away. I'd ask myself if I felt sick, if I felt crampy, if I was more tired than usual. To all of those questions, the honest answer was no. But during the next couple of weeks after the test, I became very, very cold, all the time. I couldn't get warm, no matter how many jumpers I was wearing or how high the central heating was on. I remember telling myself, 'You've just pumped yourself full of hormones, you've been through a really hard time, and now you've finally got the result you want, it's just a reaction to all that. It'll be fine.' I don't know if feeling so cold meant anything, but I later wondered whether it was my body's way of telling me something wasn't right.

Soon though, I began to worry, secretly, that something was wrong. The pregnancy tests I used then were the digital ones that tell you how far along you are from the date of conception, and no test I did ever put me at further than two to three weeks. Even when I was over five weeks, the tests never showed this. So I stopped doing them – I was frightened of what they meant and wanted to believe the best. I decided to accept that I was pregnant, not probe too much further, and wait for the scan at seven weeks. I got back into the awful habit of googling everything, which, depending on what I read, either comforted or panicked me completely. I was slowly losing the happy, positive person I had become.

On the day of the results of my blood test, Chantal had planned for us to go on a spa day together, to a beautiful place outside London. We were going to have lunch and spend the whole day there, and I'd been looking forward to it so much. On the way, though, I got a phone call from Dr Ram to say that there was something peculiar about the blood test result: it showed me as not pregnant. He said he thought the lab might have tested the wrong hormone, and that he'd look into it further and ring me back.

It did turn out that the blood test the lab had done was not the usual one where the hCG hormone is tested. This was a laboratory in London, not the clinic. To be honest, it was all very odd. But by then I was so desperately worried I had to go home; I just wouldn't have enjoyed the spa and

I wanted to be with Harry. Of course Chunny understood, so we drove home.

The next day I had another blood test, which checked the hCG levels this time and showed that I was indeed pregnant, although the levels of the hormone were low. That in itself wasn't a cause for concern – hCG starts low and rises steadily through the first trimester of a pregnancy. I could have asked for blood tests every few days, to check these levels and see if they were rising the way they should, but I didn't want to go down that road. I'd never wanted to get into that degree of monitoring – I felt that surely I was entitled to a little magic in falling pregnant, that all the checking and monitoring was done with. I needed to hope and trust. But it turned out that was difficult to do.

During the two weeks of waiting, I hadn't given much thought to how I would actually feel if the result was positive. I'd been so focused on getting pregnant that I hadn't thought at all about how I'd feel once I was. It was totally surreal to even think the words 'I'm pregnant', and in a way I felt worse knowing I was than I had done in the weeks leading up to the test. Once the initial burst of joy had calmed down, it began to sink in how delicate a thing this pregnancy was. I grew petrified, wondering if everything was going to be OK.

At the end of December, the day after the seven-week scan, Harry and I were due to go on holiday with his parents to Antigua. We'd booked it so that we would have something to look forward to either way: if the embryo didn't take hold, a holiday might cheer us up, and if it had, we thought it would be a lovely way to celebrate. I began to worry terribly about going. I was very protective of myself at that time and very anxious about taking care of our precious baby – I didn't want to do anything that could possibly do any harm to it. I began saying to Harry, 'I don't think we should go, I don't think I should fly or be away from home.' I was scared about using suncream and mosquito repellent because of the chemicals they can contain, and began researching products I could use that would be safe. I remember asking my doctor all sorts of questions – about symptoms, sunscreen, things I should and shouldn't do – I spent those long days waiting, anxiously, for the scan and for pregnancy symptoms to start.

11

Emptiness

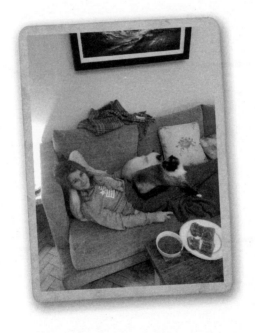

I CONTINUED TO FEEL very cold over the next few weeks. In bed at night I'd have my socks on and a woolly hat, as well as the electric blanket. It wasn't that I felt ill, I just couldn't get warm. I tried to stay in the zone of daily meditation, walks and positive affirmations but it was difficult. I was constantly on Google, checking my symptoms, or lack thereof, and my adrenaline levels were very high. I felt frazzled and anxious. It was a big change in mood from the way I'd felt during IVF.

Christmas is always a busy time for us. On top of the day itself, our wedding anniversary is 21 December and Harry's birthday is the 23rd, so it's a very full and happy time. I love the cosiness: the cold nights, the sparkly lights, being with my family. But that year I didn't want to be travelling all over the place, seeing people and being busy.

Really, all I wanted to do was stay at home, curl up by the fire with the cats, and just sleep and eat. I don't know if I'd have felt like that had I fallen pregnant naturally – maybe it was because of everything we'd gone through, and how precious our embryo was. Maybe I felt more protective. Also, there was the fact that Harry wasn't allowing himself to be excited. I wasn't feeling it from him, which I think meant that everything just felt particularly delicate and fragile.

My family has certain Christmas traditions – as every family does. As children, we always spent Christmas Day with our cousins on my mum's side. They'd usually come to us in the morning, then my brothers, being choristers, would go and sing in the chapel at King's.

Dad and my brothers still go to the Christmas Day service at King's, but Mum finds it too upsetting to go since Rupert's accident. Hearing the choristers singing brings back so many memories from when the boys were little and listening to the music is too emotional for her, so she and I stay at home and make sandwiches. Then, when everyone is back, after a late lunch there's present opening and we finally have Christmas dinner at about 10 o'clock at night.

Harry always joins in with these traditions and that Christmas was no different, except he and I decided it would be romantic to go and stay for a few nights at the place we got married, St Michael's Manor, near my family home. Because I was pregnant, he wanted me to be comfortable, and because my parents' house would be so full with all the family staying, we'd have been sleeping on a blow-up bed there. It was lovely. We checked in on Harry's birthday and had a wonderful Christmas.

I woke very early on Boxing Day, maybe 4 a.m., with a shaft of light coming in through a gap in the curtains. I went to the loo, half asleep, not really thinking about anything, but when I wiped I could see by that little bit of light that there was quite a lot of blood on the tissue.

I froze. Panic surged through me. Although I didn't want to, I forced myself to turn on the light. I knew it was important to see clearly and yes, there was a lot of blood. As I got back into bed and woke Harry, I realized how strange it feels when the person who would usually hold your hand during a difficult time is so deeply affected by it themselves; when the person who would usually embrace you and reassure you needs their own reassurance.

It was too early to ring Dr Ram and there was nothing I could do except lie quietly and try to stay calm. I wasn't in any pain or discomfort. After a while I went online and read that bleeding in early pregnancy is very common. It can be caused by a number of different things, including burst blood vessels around the cervix, and isn't necessarily a sign of impending miscarriage. I listened to my relaxation tracks and focused on staying calm. I told myself, 'There's no way I'm going to lose this baby. I've seen this embryo, it's a good embryo, this isn't going to happen. This isn't how our story goes. It's not fair, it can't be.' I didn't believe that life could be so cruel.

Usually when I have an anxiety attack, the moment the adrenaline starts pumping, my legs shake wildly and there's nothing I can do to stop them. When Harry's there, he physically holds them down, to still them so that the shaking stops. That morning, after the surge of adrenaline, I calmed myself but my legs shook uncontrollably for ages. Harry pinned them down and we finally got through it and managed to get back to sleep.

Later that morning I texted Ram. Even though it was Boxing Day he rang straight back, bless him, and said, 'Let's just keep an eye on this for the next twenty-four hours. Bleeding is common at this stage of pregnancy.' Which was reassuring. Then I rang Chantal. 'I had the same thing,' she said. 'Try not to worry. Have faith that everything will be fine.' We then went over to Mum and Dad's, and I told Mum what had happened, but I also told her what the doctor had said, what Chantal had said, and that I was sure everything was OK.

After that I had no more bleeding, so we began to feel more confident. We spent that day at my parents' and it was lovely, although every time I went to the loo I was terrified. But as the hours wore on and there was still no more blood, I began to feel more relaxed.

I was just over six weeks pregnant but I still had no real pregnancy symptoms to speak of. I had an app on my phone that told me each day what should be happening at that stage. It said that by now I might have started to feel sick, have sore breasts or experience food aversions. I felt none of these things. I knew very well that some women don't feel anything, or their symptoms are completely different to the usual ones, but I badly wanted to feel something out of the ordinary. I wanted some kind of further proof that I was pregnant. It occurred to me that my mum had been five months pregnant with Rupert before she found out – she'd stopped taking the Pill and just assumed her periods hadn't come back. So I wondered whether I was like her, one of the lucky few who escape the symptoms.

The next day, the 27th, Harry and I travelled with the rest of my family to Wiltshire, to visit my cousins. There hadn't been any more bleeding but I still found that going to the loo made me feel horribly anxious. By then I knew I just had to get through a few more days, because our first scan was booked for 29 December, the day before we were due to leave for Antigua.

I adore being with my cousins and even though they and I grew up more like sisters, Harry and I had decided to only tell immediate family we'd been going through IVF. Also, we wanted to experience that moment when, after the twelve-week scan, we surprised everyone with our announcement and showed them our ultrasound picture, just like other couples do. In hindsight, though, I feel that perhaps not telling them at that point added more strain to the situation, and I'd have felt better if it had all just been out in the open. It's hard to pretend you're fine and be your usual self when you're not feeling that way at all.

We spent one night in Wiltshire and the following day went for a pub lunch together. During the meal, I just didn't feel right and kept going to the loo to check everything was OK. I was desperate to leave and on the way home to London in the car, I began to feel pain, like period pain, which became more and more intense and uncomfortable. Harry was driving and I was sitting beside him, googling, telling him that cramping can be a normal symptom of early pregnancy. By this stage, I think he knew that something was wrong and that I was clutching at the best possible explanations, trying to persuade myself that everything would be OK. Neither of us could admit yet what we really knew was happening, not to ourselves or to each other.

I was six weeks and four days pregnant. Another woman might not even have known she was pregnant by then, so what happened next could have seemed like a late, heavy period. But I'd been on such a long journey to get pregnant that I was acutely aware of everything.

I had seen that life. I had watched as it was put inside me. I had the photo of our embryo by my bed. Everything I had done to get there, to that point, was with me in those moments. I knew exactly how long that life had been there, down to the very minute. I had done all that, and I was still failing. Or at least that's what it felt like to me – that I was failing to hold on to this life; failing to make a safe place for it and to keep it within me.

By the time we got home I was in a lot of pain and bleeding pretty constantly. It wasn't very heavy, but the blood was getting progressively darker and richer. I texted my doctor, who replied to say, 'Hang in there, Izzy. I'll see you in the morning.' But I accepted at that point that we were losing our baby. I had to accept it because I couldn't stop it – there was no one I could call, nothing I could do, no medication I could take to keep this from happening. There's such a cruel inevitability about a miscarriage, about the way in which it can't be stopped. You can't hold on to the one thing you want so badly to keep.

I felt very unwell by then: miserable, achy, sore. Harry helped me to get as comfortable as possible on the sofa, and made me some tomato soup and toast with Marmite. What else do we eat when we feel unwell, except soup and toast? He lit the fire and put on the TV, and both my cats, Murphy and Morris, came and sat with me, Murphy on my stomach and Morris beside me. They don't *ever* sit next to each other without hissing, and don't even much like to be in the same room together, but that evening they sat quietly, together, with me.

The Winnie-the-Pooh bear I've had since I was a little girl was with me too. I knew it was a case of waiting it out; of sitting and trying to be comfortable any way I could. What I really wanted was a hot-water bottle, but even then I couldn't allow myself to have one because the heat would've been bad for the baby. Really, I knew what was happening – that I was having a miscarriage – but still I held on to the desperate hope that it was all going to be OK. For the same reason, I didn't take painkillers either, although my back ached terribly. Knowing what I know now, I recognize that those pains were similar to those of very early labour.

Despite clinging to that shred of hope and doing what my doctor told me to by hanging in there, I also had the overwhelming feeling that I needed to do one last thing for this soul, this life inside me. I knew that I needed to let it pass, peacefully, so rather than fighting, tensing up and holding on, I tried to relax and accept that what would be, would be. I tried to let it go, and wish it on its way with love. After everything we'd been through, after seeing the embryo on the screen and watching as it was put inside me, it was so hard, but I believed that I had to. I had invested in it, believed in it, loved it, but now I needed to say goodbye.

As well as wanting to let go peacefully, I also felt so sorry for our baby, for me and for us. 'How is that fair?' I wondered. 'Why me? Why us? How do I not deserve a break?' Harry had been such a rock through everything. He'd taken care of us as best he could, and I felt it was so unfair on him too. I could see he was in just as much pain as I was.

We went to bed and the pain continued. That night was incredibly spiritual, though. I felt as if I was on a different planet. A tiny part of me still continued to hope but deep down I knew I was losing the baby, and there was something that made me feel very connected to what was happening. It was as if I was setting something free, even though I wanted to keep it so much.

Although the pain was constant and unrelenting, I finally fell asleep around 3 a.m. I woke about three hours later and again the cats were with me. I realized I was no longer in pain and wondered for a moment whether everything was actually OK and I wasn't miscarrying after all. Harry went downstairs to make breakfast and I got up. I found it really difficult to stand up – I was incredibly dizzy – but the pain had definitely stopped. Still there was that little part of me that couldn't stop hoping.

Emptiness

I went to the loo and it was then that I felt the sensation of the baby passing through me and out into the loo. I felt our little soul leave me, a physical feeling I will never forget. There, lying helpless, all our hopes and dreams. How were we supposed to flush them away? It was a feeling so cold and terrifying, so utterly lonely – the sensation of losing something so precious – it will never leave me.

I shouted downstairs to Harry, 'We've lost it! We've lost it. It's gone.' He ran upstairs. I couldn't look. I left the bathroom. There was no way I was going to flush. I didn't know at all what to do. What do you do in such a terrible situation? I know that Harry later took charge of everything, making decisions that no one should ever have to make.

We went to the scan that morning. It had been meant to be such an exciting moment – we'd wondered whether we would see a heartbeat, what the baby would look like, whether we'd be able to make out anything on the screen. Instead we got into the car and the silence between us was deafening. The journey I'd been so excited about making was now a cold nightmare. We sat quietly yet the love we have for each other filled the car loudly. In those moments, there seemed to be nothing more for either of us to say or do. I couldn't begin to think, 'What next?' I knew, and had accepted, what had happened but I still needed proof from my doctor.

When we got there, I said to Ram, 'I don't want to look at the screen.' So I didn't, although Harry did. 'I'm afraid, Izzy, that you have lost the baby,' Ram told us.

Gone, alone, empty … He tried to make the best of

it, telling me that I wouldn't need a D&C (dilation and curettage, which is a procedure done after a miscarriage to remove pregnancy tissue from inside the uterus, to clear the uterine lining), that everything had been expelled naturally and I wouldn't need to go into hospital.

I think because he'd been along the path with me and Harry, Ram felt sorry for us. 'Have a holiday, and we'll meet when you come back,' he said. 'There's nothing we can do until the bleeding has stopped, and that can take up to six weeks.'

We went home, both still very quiet, and when we arrived we found a pigeon had flown into the window of our conservatory and died. By the strangest coincidence, I'd seen the exact same thing once before when I was staying at my parents' house, on the day my mother's sister died of ovarian cancer. It was really haunting, and even now I worry about seeing dead pigeons. They make me terrified that something bad will happen.

By then, I felt completely cold and empty. I guess it was like I was outside my body, looking in as the day unfolded like an awful nightmare. It was by far the bleakest day I've ever experienced: dark and lonely. The atmosphere was so dreary and depressing, it was just awful. Harry and I took it in turns to hold each other and cry. We never fully let go together, because one of us was always trying to be strong for the other. In a situation like that, when your soulmate, the person who is usually there to support you, feels the same loss and grief, there's nothing to do but try to help each other, even as you process your own sadness.

Emptiness

That day I had a feeling of overwhelming empathy for my parents and the grief they must have experienced following Rupert's accident. I couldn't get the thought out of my head. How did they continue to get up each morning and carry on with life, let alone stay as strong as they did for the rest of us? I suddenly felt a deeper understanding of their loss. While I knew that I was facing my own grief that day, I also knew that as time passed it would get easier. Of course I wouldn't ever forget what had happened, but I would heal. It suddenly dawned on me that my parents would never escape their grief. The admiration I felt for their love for one another was immense and their unbelievable strength was an inspiration.

Harry and I rang our families to tell them the news. My brother Magnus and his wife, Marije, were still in Wiltshire at my cousins' but they got in their car straight away and drove up to London to be with us. Dad came over to our house, too, but Mum didn't as she wasn't feeling well – I think due to worry and upset. She didn't know how to deal with what was happening – she'd been with me every step of the way but there was nothing she could do to make it better. A mother's love. We are so connected that she was physically ill at the thought of what I was going through.

I remember once saying to her that I wanted a baby for her as well, for the family, because of what had happened to Rupert. 'Izzy, all I want is for my daughter to be happy,' she'd said. 'If you didn't want children, I'd be happy with that – you're everything to me.' So it wasn't for her own sake that she was so upset that day, it was entirely for me.

She might also have felt a bit guilty because her pregnancies had happened so easily, which meant she couldn't fully empathize, and that must be very difficult for a mum. Growing up, my parents had always joked they only had to pass on the stairs and Mum was pregnant.

Along with the grief and the constant questioning of why this was so hard for me, why every hurdle was so high, I was also fearful. I wondered if, on top of everything else, the miscarriage had opened up a new issue, a new nightmare for me. That not only was it difficult for my body to conceive, but perhaps it wasn't able to carry a baby either. Perhaps I simply wasn't built for this.

Had I tempted fate by having IVF, by interfering with nature and forcing a result – was this my judgement for that? Was this the universe telling me that I had to back off and accept that the answer, for me, was always going to be no? I knew in my heart that wasn't true but still, in that moment, I needed to blame something, and again I chose to blame myself.

On that terrible day I was already planning ahead. Being mindful and living in the present was impossible. Half of me was thinking about what to do next and the other half was thinking that I might not have the energy for another round of IVF, to get myself in the right frame of mind to try again. I was exhausted, demoralized and felt as if I'd never be able to find the kind of positive energy I'd had for the first cycle. I felt I'd failed my baby, and failed Harry, and failed myself, and I didn't know where to go to change that.

Emptiness

I couldn't bear it when people said, 'It wasn't meant to be, something obviously wasn't right', even though I knew they meant it kindly. I didn't feel that. I know Harry found some comfort in that idea but in my mind I was the one who wasn't right. 'How can it have failed?' I thought. 'It was our highest quality embryo; it won the race. It was perfect. There was no problem with it. It's my failure.'

The next day we flew to Antigua, and we were both so happy to be getting on the plane – to the sun, to a new place away from the dark and the misery of what had happened. But there were reminders everywhere: in my bag was the suncream and mosquito repellent I'd researched and which were safe to use during pregnancy. On the way to the plane I started to get a headache, so Harry gave me a packet of painkillers. For a split second I forgot what had

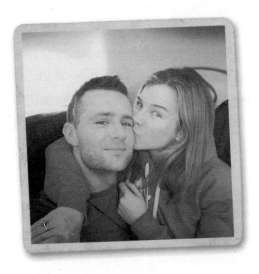

On the plane to Antigua, keen to get away from the misery of what had happened.

happened and checked to see whether they were OK to take during pregnancy.

Once on the plane, one of my legs began to throb and became uncomfortable. Me being me, I thought it was thrombosis and that I was going to die. I started crying and became very anxious, and Harry was worried too because it was really aching. We told the cabin crew, who radioed down to ground control for medical advice, and in the meantime I spoke to a very sweet member of staff. I had to tell her I'd just had a miscarriage, because that meant there was a slightly higher chance of it actually being thrombosis, and she and I got talking. It turned out that she was about to start her first round of IVF. Isn't it typical how life does that? Of all the members of crew to be working on that day, I ended up confiding in someone about to go through IVF themselves. I told her about all the holistic things I'd done and how helpful I'd found them. The thought that I could share what I had learned and that it might perhaps help someone else made me feel much better.

We got to Antigua and Harry's parents were amazing. They kept things normal, even though I'm sure they were deeply upset too. I moved between our hotel room, the restaurant and the beach every day, no further. It was perfect for what it was, and Harry and I did our best to comfort each other.

I woke up every morning to blue sky and sunshine, and yet it was like waking up the mornings following Roops' accident – to the memory of what had happened and the feeling of grief in my tummy. At first you don't remember and life is normal, then it all floods back: that sensation that something horrible has happened, even though you can't remember immediately exactly what it is.

It was hard to get out of bed and summon the energy for the day. I didn't even want to wear a bikini because I didn't like the way I looked. I'd been pumped full of hormones, I was bloated and still bleeding. The blood loss was relentless and I was desperate for it to stop. I couldn't even use tampons because my cervix might have been dilated, which carries an increased risk of infection. So it really was horrible, and a constant reminder of the awful experience.

We'd go to the beach each day and I'd take a book with me, but mostly I listened to music because I've always used

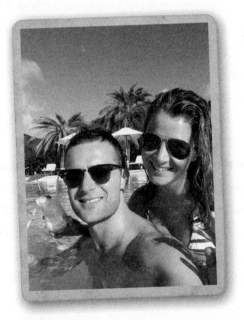

Although it was a relief to get away,
the sunshine and smiles don't reflect the pain
we were going through after the miscarriage.

it to cope with difficult periods in life. I listened to 'Quanta Qualia' so often that I'll always associate it with that time. It's such a beautiful piece of music but I find it difficult to listen to now without crying.

After the first few days Harry and I began to talk about the future. Almost immediately after we found out I was pregnant we had started discussing moving house because where we lived wasn't a family home. It was stunning, a former artist's studio with our bedroom on a mezzanine, and I adored it, but it wasn't suitable for children. Even though we didn't have any yet I still wanted to move, because I knew that if we stayed put, I'd feel absolutely stuck and as if we weren't moving forward with our plans. We wanted to find a house that needed doing up, so we could throw our energy into it. I wanted a project, something creative and new that would feel as if we were moving forward with our lives.

We looked for properties online, setting up viewings for when we got back from Antigua. Even though we were putting so much effort into thinking about a new home, I was still keen to talk to Harry about what else we might do next; when we might think about trying a second IVF cycle.

Harry was about to go to Australia on tour – McFly were supporting One Direction there – and I'd decided to go with him. My feeling was that we could get in one round of IVF before we went but Harry, thankfully, was more measured, determined to slow things down. 'Let's not think too far ahead. Let's get you mentally and physically better first,' he said to me. I'm so grateful that he took on the rational-thinking role and put the brakes on. Looking back, I wasn't ready to go ahead with a second round of IVF so soon, but at the time I believed I was.

Miscarriage is so horribly common and yes, mine happened very early on. I can't begin to think about what some women go through with a later loss. But I do know that if that's what I went through, it shows you the strength of the bond between mother and child. People can be very quick to say, 'Oh, it was so early. If you hadn't been having IVF you might not even have known you were pregnant.' But I did know, and I still mourn the loss of that baby. And I think about the knock-on effect: I wonder would Lola have been the second child if the miscarriage had never happened? And what would it have been like, for her and us, if she had had an older brother or sister? Of course these are questions that no one can ever answer, but I wondered about them then, and I sometimes wonder about them now.

I still think of that baby as my first child. I felt so connected to that embryo from the very beginning. Even during my pregnancy with Lola, I never had quite the same immediate attachment as I did the first time. Possibly because the first experience meant I never felt I could relax with Lola until she actually arrived safely. I was always so fearful of something happening that I stayed focused on reaching the next milestone, making it to the end of each week, and getting one step closer to her being safely outside my body.

Some people say that the spirit of an unborn child comes back in your next baby, which is a beautiful thought. A friend of mine said to me that what made their miscarriage a little easier to bear was the thought that if they hadn't suffered their loss, they may never have met their next baby. For me it was different because our embryos were in a pack, three of them, ready to go from the same moment. It's comforting to know that Lola was part of that, and somehow it feels as if we are all still connected to our little soul.

12

Picking up the pieces

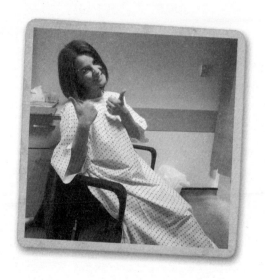

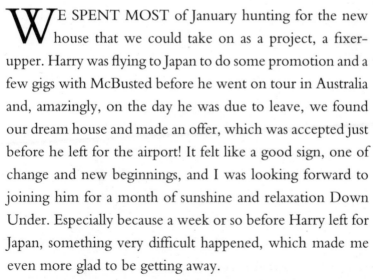

W E SPENT MOST of January hunting for the new house that we could take on as a project, a fixer-upper. Harry was flying to Japan to do some promotion and a few gigs with McBusted before he went on tour in Australia and, amazingly, on the day he was due to leave, we found our dream house and made an offer, which was accepted just before he left for the airport! It felt like a good sign, one of change and new beginnings, and I was looking forward to joining him for a month of sunshine and relaxation Down Under. Especially because a week or so before Harry left for Japan, something very difficult happened, which made me even more glad to be getting away.

My brother Magnus phoned Harry. I thought it strange that he was ringing Harry, not me, and then I heard Harry say, 'I'm sorry, Magnus, but you're going to have to tell Izzy yourself, I'm passing the phone over.' And I knew. Straight away, I knew. Sure enough, Magnus and his wife, Marije, were pregnant.

That was when the anger finally hit. Until then I'd been filled with grief, fear and regret, but not anger. I'd just been told by two of the people I loved most in the world that I was going to be an auntie, and what I felt was rage. All I could think was, 'Of course! Of course this is the next thing that happens in the story! The next thing I have to deal with!'

The two babies would have been born weeks apart, and I realized that I'd have to go through the whole of Marije's pregnancy thinking about where I would've been with my own. Once born, my niece or nephew would be almost the same age as the baby we didn't have, and everything they ever did would be a reminder of what should have been for us.

Obviously, my rational mind was fighting against these feelings, but I couldn't help my reaction at the time. I loathed myself in every possible way for having any emotion other than sheer joy for them. Magnus could not have been more sensitive. I knew he would have been stewing before making that phone call, and while he was talking to me he kept apologizing. The thought of that still breaks my heart. Then Marije – an amazing, generous, selfless person – came on the phone. She cried down the line, saying, 'I wish I wasn't,' and that was even more upsetting. Much later, she told me that for her the pregnancy felt wrong, that all she wanted to do was give me her baby, and I know she truly felt that. She has the kindest soul.

Picking up the pieces

I tried to be as delighted as possible for them, but I just had to get off the phone. It was their first month of trying for a baby and I couldn't believe that it had happened so quickly, so easily for them. I never let them know that I was feeling any of those things – I kept it all to myself.

I rang Mum then and found myself shouting down the phone to her like I'd never done before: 'How is this fair? How is it so easy for them?' It was the first time in years I heard my mum cry. I think she felt so torn – she had one child with happy news and another devastated because of it. I know she felt my pain almost as much as I did.

They were difficult days and became even worse when Marije tragically had a miscarriage at thirteen weeks. As well as feeling utterly heartbroken for her and Magnus, I also felt a huge amount of guilt, more than I'd ever experienced before. I'd dreaded having to go through their pregnancy, but when the miscarriage happened I realized how selfish I'd been for ever thinking about myself rather than them. Every pregnancy is precious, everybody needs to be loved and supported through it, but I'd been so focused on my own problems that I hadn't done enough to be there for them.

I couldn't have made any difference to what happened, of course – no one could have – but I knew neither of them had been able to relax during the pregnancy because of what had happened to me. They'd both been worried from the start.

Worst of all, I wasn't able to be there with them the night it happened. I was back from Australia by then, but on tour with Harry in Leeds. Because everything happened very late in the evening, I couldn't get to them soon enough. They'd travelled to be with me the morning of my miscarriage and I couldn't do the same when it happened to them. Marije was very ill, as she lost a lot of blood. I was on the phone to Magnus through the night but I should have been there, and that night still haunts me.

After what we both experienced, Magnus and I became even closer. He understood on a deep level what Harry and I were going through, and we just wanted to support and help each other during these difficult times in our lives. For all that Magnus had feared not being able to take over the oldest brother role from Rupert, my opinion is that he did a wonderful job of it, constantly checking up on me and making sure I was OK.

And yet, I missed Rupert so much during those months. I wondered what life might have been like if the accident had never happened; what he might have said or done to try to help. Of course he was still there as a reminder of the many ways in which I was – and am – lucky, and he brought much-needed perspective to my life.

Given everything that was going on in our lives, the trip to Australia had been just what Harry and I needed. A holiday for me, work for Harry (which he loves), sunshine, rest, a change of scenery, and a chance to put some distance between us and the sorrow we felt. Gi came on that trip too, with little Buzz, and I had great fun with her and many cuddles and giggles with him.

Georgia, Danny's wife, was also with us – she has such a great sense of humour, which kept me smiling. She and

I both enjoy exercising, so that helped me to get back on track. We'd go on runs together in the sunshine, followed by healthy smoothies, yummy lunches and plenty of chats. Both she and Gi were such a comfort to me, and always there to listen if I needed to talk. We certainly made the most of Australia's healthy, outdoorsy lifestyle and the sunshine, and Harry and I came back knowing that we were ready, psychologically, to try again.

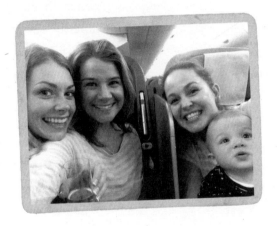

*Georgia and Gi were a huge comfort
to me on the trip to Australia.*

When we got back home, Harry had to go back on tour around the UK with McBusted. So I started on the Pill for the month, as my doctors had directed, to get ready to begin the IVF process again. Even though Australia had helped me kick-start a healthy lifestyle once more, I still found it very difficult to snap back into the mindset I'd been in first time around.

During the first cycle I'd been so proactive and positive,

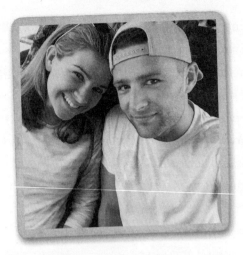

*Harry and I came home knowing we were
ready for another IVF cycle.*

whereas now I was beginning on the back of a 'failure', and that made me more worried than I'd previously been. There was so much more uncertainty, so many terrible questions in my mind, that this new round held a whole new level of pressure and fear.

I knew I needed to be in the same good health as before – this embryo deserved the same positive state of mind and body that I'd had with the first one but it was so much more difficult to get into that space this time. This was mainly because I wasn't at home and therefore not in my usual routine. Being away and touring, it was so much harder to cook food I knew was full of goodness and had the right nutrients in it, as I'd been able to do the last time around. On tour, you're eating out in restaurants, often at strange times to fit in with the band's schedule, plus there's a lot of moving about, with different hotel rooms every night.

Picking up the pieces

Once the tour finished and we were home and settled, I worked hard to get back into the right frame of mind. I centred myself again, and focused on myself and my body, instead of being distracted by travel, the new house and our renovation plans. I went back on the nutrition plan – the green smoothies and beetroot risottos – back to walking, swimming, yoga and lots of fresh air.

I mentioned to Gi that I was struggling to get my head back to the place it had been in, so she recommended I meet a friend of hers called Hollie de Cruz, who teaches hypnobirthing. Of course I wasn't ready for hypnobirthing – yet – but she came to my house and did some hypnotherapy with me, to help me stay calm and focused. Sure enough, a few sessions with Hollie helped me feel so much better. She has such an amazing presence – she only has to step into the room and you feel calmer. Once you've been to that place of tranquillity and done all the practice, it becomes like a muscle memory, a state of mind you can access again quite quickly. Soon, I felt ready to go once more.

After the sessions with Hollie, and about three months after the miscarriage, I felt that I'd cleared my mind and was ready for the next round. The second time was all very different. By then Harry and I were living in a sweet, rented one-bedroom flat nearby because the house we'd bought and were doing up wasn't yet ready to move into. Being in the flat felt like a fresh start because there were no associations with what had happened. Also, it was early spring, a time of new beginnings and, perhaps most importantly, I began to feel differently about what had happened to me, and about what might happen next.

I'd survived the miscarriage. Terrible as it had been, I'd got through it. That made me realize I had more strength maybe than I knew. I felt as if I was in a good place. At the back of my mind, I'd started to believe that even if it didn't happen on this occasion, it *was* going to happen. I learned to stop myself putting all my expectations onto the next round of IVF and concentrated on the positives instead: 'I've fallen pregnant before. My body can do this. Even if it doesn't happen this time, it *will* happen. I'm young, it's all in my favour. It can happen.'

With all this in mind, I felt strong enough to move forward.

With this cycle, Harry and I were far more open with the people around us. Partly because we felt, and still feel, that there shouldn't be any shame or secrecy around IVF, but also because we'd learned how much support you need when something bad happens. If you do miscarry, you really need the love of family and friends to help you through. Knowing that as I did, there was no question of me not telling. I also didn't want the added pressure of feeling that I was keeping secrets from anyone.

I didn't have to prepare my body in quite the same way this time. There would be no stimulation phase and egg collection, which I had been so nervous about last time, because I already had the two frozen embryos in storage. As a result I wasn't scanned as regularly during those first two weeks, and so didn't have the injections and scan appointments to focus on. I just had to sit back and hope that my womb lining was thickening (back to the beetroot risottos!) and that my ovaries were nice and quiet – it made a change to want to see quiet ovaries!

Early in my frozen embryo transfer (FET) cycle, I started taking the medication Progynova, an oestrogen tablet which is needed to help thicken your womb lining ready for the embryo transfer, and to maintain the lining should the embryo implant successfully. You also take a low dose of aspirin with Progynova to reduce the small risk of thrombosis.

I'd told my doctor that I wanted to be treated like someone who had had recurrent miscarriages, by which I mean that I wanted more interventions than would usually be recommended following one miscarriage. Clinics vary on this but some will only increase dosages or prescribe extra drugs after three miscarriages, and I had no intention of waiting for that to happen to me. Even though I knew that miscarriage is very common and there wasn't any evidence to suggest that I had particular problems, I didn't want to go through it again. I wanted to do everything I could to give myself the best possible chance of a successful pregnancy.

Dr Ram started me on a drug called Clexane, which is like a stronger form of aspirin and helps to thin the blood – one of the most common causes of miscarriage is blood-clotting disorders. Alongside the same dosage of aspirin that I'd taken the first time around, I took the Clexane in the form of a daily injection into my tummy area, which gave me awful bruises. I also had the pipelle procedure carried out again, where they irritate the lining of the womb.

Dare to dream

At the start of our second round Harry and I discussed with the doctors whether both embryos would be transferred, meaning that I could end up carrying twins. That was a bit of an 'oh my goodness' moment, especially for Harry! As we'd only had one embryo transferred the first time, the idea of this was a bit of a shock.

IVF protocols change all the time, and they vary from woman to woman. Sometimes the doctors feel that the success rate from a frozen embryo is slightly lower than from a fresh one, and therefore implanting two gives a higher chance of at least one being carried to full term. But on the other hand, if neither implants, then you've lost both embryos in one go, and in my case that would've meant having no more insurance, no last fertilized embryo in the freezer. Ultimately, based on my age and the fact that I fell pregnant with the first cycle, the doctors recommended against transferring two embryos, so we trusted their decision. But not before Harry and I spent a crazy few days wondering how on earth we might cope if we had twins!

Once the lining of my womb had thickened enough, it was time to do the transfer. The frozen embryo isn't thawed until the day of the transfer itself, and sometimes things can go wrong during the thawing process. We understood the risks and felt comforted that we still had a third and final embryo, believing that surely one of the two would be OK. Luckily for us, this amazing little embryo made it.

On the morning of 29 April 2015, the call came through while we were sat in the same old coffee shop near our flat, killing time and waiting to learn our fate. I answered the phone and when I heard the news, a huge smile beamed across my face. I don't think I realized how nervous I'd been until I felt the relief that everything was OK, and that our little frozen embryo had made it. Again we were one step closer.

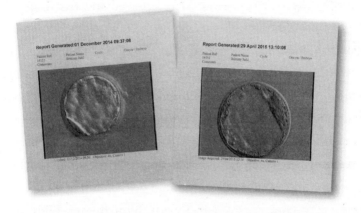

Harry and I felt very lucky to have the chance to see our two beautiful embryos. Both times it was the most magical moment for us during IVF treatment.

We raced to the car, drove to the clinic, and there we were again, back in the same sterile transfer room. Out came the new embryo, and to our surprise it looked nothing like the first. Even though it looked like another beautiful full moon, it had a completely different structure, which fascinated us. 'That's a girl,' Harry said. I told him not to be silly – how could he tell? – but of course he was right.

The transfer was just as magical as the first time. Again we watched as the embryo was placed inside me, and we saw the flash of light as it was released. I felt calm and positive, happy that another beautiful embryo was back home where it belonged. Once the transfer was done, I had just a week to wait rather than two – which was the protocol at Herts & Essex with a frozen embryo transfer – then I was to go back in for a blood test to find out if I was pregnant. I was so grateful not to have to pee on any more sticks.

The second time around everything felt familiar and much easier. I knew I was going to be taking the progesterone in the form that suited me better, I was pleased to be doing a blood test at the clinic and getting the results there and then (because of what had happened the first time when the London laboratory had done the blood test), and this time I only had a week to wait, not two.

I was desperate for this cycle to work, of course I was, but not in the same way as I had been the first time. Getting a positive pregnancy test result was just one part of the process. First time around, I believed that once I'd got the result I wanted, everything else would take care of itself. This time, I knew that getting pregnant would just be the beginning and there was so much more to come after that. I knew I needed to pace myself, to save my energy.

The seventh of May was the date of the blood test. Harry and I went to the clinic together in the morning, they took my blood, and then we had to wait around half an hour. It was torture. I think Harry was feeling worse than me – he was pacing up and down – so I suggested that we go outside for a walk. In reality, the walk probably lasted all of three minutes, because when we came back we found we still had twenty minutes left to kill! Finally, the nurse arrived with our results, but we had the agony of yet another wait while we cleared the security questions she was obliged to ask us first.

Only then did she tell us that our result was positive. I just couldn't believe it. 'No, no, it can't be. No way!' I said. I felt huge relief, followed by an instant memory of the miscarriage and how we had a long way to go yet. Harry and I were very cautious about celebrating – we just breathed a sigh of relief at the fact that we were over yet another hurdle. It wasn't the way I ever thought we'd react to a positive pregnancy test!

We'd planned to go to Suffolk and see Harry's parents that day. They live in a beautiful, peaceful part of the countryside and we wanted to have something comforting to do that morning, no matter what happened. They knew where we'd been, so we were able to tell them the wonderful news straight away.

I've always thought about how much I'd have loved to have been able to get to twelve weeks pregnant and announce the happy news to our families out of the blue. That just wasn't how it was for us, though. Our families were deeply involved from the very start but that was something beautiful in its own right.

As we went through this second pregnancy it meant so much to me and Harry to know that they were all with us, supporting us and willing it to be successful.

13

Daring to dream

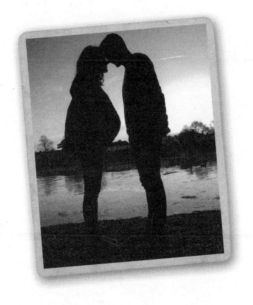

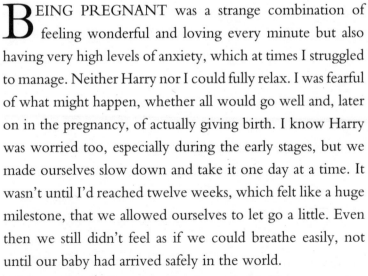

B EING PREGNANT was a strange combination of feeling wonderful and loving every minute but also having very high levels of anxiety, which at times I struggled to manage. Neither Harry nor I could fully relax. I was fearful of what might happen, whether all would go well and, later on in the pregnancy, of actually giving birth. I know Harry was worried too, especially during the early stages, but we made ourselves slow down and take it one day at a time. It wasn't until I'd reached twelve weeks, which felt like a huge milestone, that we allowed ourselves to let go a little. Even then we still didn't feel as if we could breathe easily, not until our baby had arrived safely in the world.

Just getting to the end of each week felt like an eternity, but in some ways it was more difficult for Harry than it was for me, I think. I guess when you're feeling dreadful during early pregnancy, you at least know that your body is changing and doing things and working. Harry just had to wait it out.

At around six weeks, we were due to have a scan. I could have had blood tests before that, to check that my hCG levels were rising as they should be, but I chose not to. In many ways, I was much more practical and less emotional the second time around. This was partly my way of protecting myself, but it was also because I'd now fallen pregnant twice. Knowing I'd done so made me relax a bit, because I knew it could happen. I was so grateful that the cycle hadn't failed, and that we had the opportunity to try again, if necessary, with the third embryo that was waiting for us in the freezer. I really thank my lucky stars for that.

Also, by about six weeks, I felt awful. Really tired and as sick as a dog – and never was I happier. Every day that I felt rotten, I celebrated, because it meant that I actually was feeling pregnant. I had the symptoms I should have had and, despite how unwell I felt, that was very reassuring.

The flat we were renting was tiny, and the cooking smells from the kitchen used to really bother me. I remember being under the covers in bed, trying to hide, without success! Even the scent of clean laundry made me feel nauseous.

When I felt like I could eat, I just craved stodge – bread and pasta mainly – and I made the most of it. It was the one time in my life that I didn't give my body a hard time. I ate little and often, and all the things I usually didn't want to eat. Having been so healthy while on my fertility nutrition plan, I felt bad for not continuing in that vein but I couldn't stomach the green smoothies – I just trusted that my body was telling me what it needed.

I also had terrible headaches during the first trimester, really pounding ones. On one occasion, I remember sitting at home watching Wimbledon with a pair of sunglasses on, the fan going full blast, and an ice pack on my head. I was afraid to take even one paracetamol, despite it being safe to do so during pregnancy.

I felt really nervous before our early scan because our last experience had been so terrible and sad. We weren't expecting to hear the heartbeat – at that stage it wouldn't have been unusual not to – but at five weeks and four days, we did. As I lay there, with Harry beside me, the sound of Lola's heart came to us loud and clear. We couldn't believe it. The thought that I had two beating hearts, mine and hers, totally amazed me. It's so beautiful to think that Lola knows what my heart sounds like from inside my body! It's difficult to describe the overwhelming emotion of that moment – the hope of new life, the first time we heard our baby. Harry recorded it on his phone and we listened to it over and over again during those early months.

Despite the reassurance from our early scan and hearing Lola's heartbeat, getting beyond six weeks and four days was still very much on my mind. That was when my first pregnancy had ended. Despite everything feeling different this time, I knew that this milestone was looming ahead of both of us. On the date itself we were visiting Harry's grandmother, who still lives in the house she grew up in, a beautiful old mill. We were staying in a cosy room with two single beds, from which we could hear the soothing sound of the water outside.

The night itself was a long one. I was up and down to the loo constantly, checking and checking again that there was no bleeding. I was very, very anxious, and so afraid of what might happen, wondering how we would possibly cope if something did. When morning came and all was still well, I felt as if a huge obstacle was finally behind me.

I continued to take the extra progesterone, the aspirin and the Clexane until sixteen weeks – most women will only take them until twelve weeks – and even then I was really scared to stop. The feeling I got once I did, though, was amazing. I was so excited, thinking, 'I'm finally doing this by myself! My body is doing this all alone!' Every day that followed, because I knew my body was doing its job, I felt a real sense of confidence: I was now growing our baby by myself, with no help from anyone or anything. It had been a bit like learning to ride a bike with someone holding on to you at first. Then comes the wonderful moment when they let go and you realize you're pedalling all by yourself!

Another piece of happy news we received around this time was that Magnus and Marije had fallen pregnant again a month after we did, so our daughters, Lola and Alma, were born just a month apart. Magnus and Marije believe this is the way it was always supposed to be – that I was meant to have the first baby and they were meant to have the second. I don't know if that's so, but it's lovely for all of us that the two girls are so close in age.

On top of that early ultrasound, I had a few more scans

during the pregnancy than would be usual, and to some extent they helped to keep my anxiety at bay. It did flare up on occasion though, which I think was partly due to the changes in my hormones, and partly because I was feeling so nervous about giving birth. I also had overwhelming moments of realization that when our baby was born, he or she was going to be completely dependent on us, twenty-four seven.

I know this seems obvious, but when you sometimes wonder whether you're even able to take care of yourself, you question whether you're strong enough to take care of a tiny little bundle. I worried about whether I'd be able to cope with the responsibility but also felt terribly guilty for even having those thoughts and anxieties in the first place, after all we'd gone through. Having longed to be pregnant, I felt I should be nothing but grateful, and owed it to all the couples who longed to be in our position. I'm sure guilt is a very normal emotion to experience but it's something I still have to work on – I have to remind myself that it's OK to have bad days.

I've also learned that anxieties and fears never disappear – there will always be another worry. In fact I'm sure this is the lesson I was meant to learn from all this: don't cross bridges until you come to them. We can't be in control of everything. Surely when you experience something difficult in your life, there's always a greater lesson to come from it?

We chose not to find out if we were having a boy or a girl. Every single other thing about the pregnancy had been planned and organized and monitored, so it was the one thing I felt we could leave as a surprise. It was important to both me and Harry that we didn't know, that some degree of mystery should remain.

As time went on, I grew increasingly terrified of giving birth naturally, of being out of control, and of something happening to the baby or me. I was fine with the idea of pain, but fearful of not knowing what to expect. I became so frightened, an elective Caesarean section began to seem like a good idea. I reasoned that if I had a C-section, everything would be planned and under control. Everyone who needed to be there would be present and nothing unpredictable would happen. I had it all worked out.

When I mentioned the idea to Harry he was – as he always is – very calm and rational. He didn't put any pressure on me either way. He just said, 'If that's what you want, I'll support you, but why don't we wait and see how you feel? We don't need to make any decisions yet.'

Before long I'd talked myself into it. Then, one day, Mum was over for lunch and I told her how nervous I was. Apparently she'd felt a similar fear about giving birth to Rupert, her first baby. She was so scared that she asked to be induced. She'd never told me that before, but it showed me that even though Mum and I are different in many ways, there are clearly things we have in common. 'But I wouldn't have done it four times if it had been that bad,' she said. 'You'll be fine, it's magical.' Her words comforted me hugely and from that day I felt much more confident about managing my anxieties around a natural birth.

Harry and I also decided that seeing the lovely Hollie

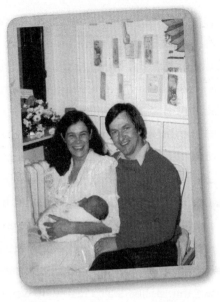

*My mum had felt as nervous as I did about
giving birth – but reassured me that she wouldn't
have done it four times had it been that bad!*

de Cruz again would help with my fears. She guided us through a brilliant hypnobirthing course that included visualizations and meditations for pregnancy, labour and birth. It was a lot more practical than I'd expected it to be: Hollie explains exactly what happens physically in your body as you labour and deliver your baby. She also gave us a copy of *The Hypnobirthing Book* by Katharine Graves, which, along with Hollie's audios, completely changed the way I thought about birth.

I suppose having done a lot of mindfulness and visualizations throughout my detox and IVF cycles, I soon realized I had all the necessary tools to tap into a calm state of mind and remain there. I started to understand how it was important to keep practising and prepare as best I could for the big day.

The other great thing about hypnobirthing is that it gave Harry a role to play. As well as being the person to read the guided meditations to me during pregnancy, Hollie also asked him to put up positive affirmations about birth around the flat. He chose to stick 'I am a strong and confident woman' on the front door, which made us laugh and entertained anyone who came to visit! Hollie also made practical suggestions about what he could do to help during the birth. He packed the hospital bag so that he knew where everything was, he reminded me of the breathing techniques I needed to use, he fuelled me with energy snacks, was my TENS machine hero, and generally my absolute rock.

I may have learned a lot about remaining calm, but pretty much from the start of my pregnancy, baby brain kicked in. I went from being the most organized person in the world to sending me and Harry to the wrong airport! We were on our way to Heathrow to go on holiday when I remembered that actually, we were meant to be flying from Gatwick. Harry kept wondering, 'Where's my organized wife gone?' He even had to take over most of the planning for our house renovations, something I'd have thrown myself into usually, but all I could focus on was the baby!

Me and my baby brain still enjoyed indulging in my interests and hobbies. I carried on playing my violin and it was during a concert that I felt Lola kick for the first time. It took my breath away and the world felt like it stopped for a few seconds. It is such a beautiful moment and, for me, the first time I truly bonded with Lola. To feel her move made it all so real. I didn't care that we were in the middle of a performance, I wanted to shout out and tell the world I'd just felt my baby kick for the first time. It felt like the start of all the many memories we would share together, just the two of us. The concert I was playing in was a particularly emotional one even before the kick happened – it was at a classical music festival in Hatfield, organized by my brother Guy, and we were performing with the choir from King's. Also, the conductor was Stephen Cleobury, who had conducted at King's back when all my brothers were choristers there.

Almost more amazing was the first time that Harry felt Lola kicking. We were watching Take That at The O2 so I couldn't hear a word he said but I'll never forget the look on his face when I put his hand on my tummy!

I didn't really read any pregnancy books – I just wanted to trust my instincts and figure things out for myself. I was also nervous about looking too far ahead. In the last couple of weeks before Lola was due, there was one book I did read, about breastfeeding. Many people had said to me how breastfeeding can be a challenge, so I felt it might be helpful to prepare for that.

By the time Lola was born, I was nine days overdue. Despite my great efforts to remain calm, my anxiety crept up on me as the due date grew closer. I don't think I could relax enough to let my body get into the swing of what it needed to do – too much stress can cause labour to slow down or even stall it completely. Either that or Lola was just too comfy where she was and not ready to make an appearance yet. I tried all the tricks, including eating copious amounts of pineapple, drinking endless cups of raspberry leaf tea and bouncing on my birth ball. My favourite was indulging in the most relaxing reflexology, thanks to a lovely local reflexologist called Lulu!

In the end I asked my midwives if I could be induced, because I just wanted to get started. I found both the waiting and anticipation made me feel worse, but the midwives were reluctant, as was Harry – again being the rational one. They all wanted to give me a little longer. Eventually I had a sweep when I was eight days past my due date and sure enough I went into labour that night.

About 3 a.m. I had a show and the contractions started. At first, they were regular and slow, and I could cope fine. Once I'm immersed in a situation, I'm much better. It's always the anticipation of something that is worse for me. So for the first few hours of labour, I was really in the zone. All the preparation I had done with hypnobirthing kicked in and I even enjoyed it. I felt that I was in control and ready for it.

We left for the hospital at about 4 a.m. – I'd had a little more bleeding than normal with my show so the midwives suggested I come in. By the time we got there the contractions were regular and strong, I was checked over by the doctor and all was well. I had with me my granny's hankie with lavender oil on it, a playlist of music I loved, and my affirmations dotted throughout the room. Hollie had kindly made my favourite one into an A4 poster – it read 'all is calm, all is well, I am safe'.

Once labour became quite intense, I couldn't get

comfortable anywhere other than draped over a birthing ball. Harry was on the floor in front of me with the TENS machine, controlling the boost. I found listening to music comforting and on my playlist I had a recording of the piece of music that my brothers Guy and Magnus had performed as I walked up the aisle on our wedding day – 'Gabriel's Oboe'– and that version of them playing it came on between contractions.

The piece lasted for the exact period between two strong contractions and although Ali, our midwife, was there, she said nothing. It felt like it was just Harry and me, alone in the world together while the beautiful music filled the room. We locked eyes and didn't say a word. We just stayed like that for the length of the piece. I know we both had such lovely memories of our wedding day. And I think we both knew that those were our last moments together, just the two of us. It was magical. A chance to communicate silently to each other, 'We're in this together.' I felt so much love.

After that, the contractions went off the scale and I transitioned from this lovely, calm place to questioning if I had the strength to carry on. I remember an overwhelming feeling of exhaustion and a sense of being out of control. It felt like my mind couldn't keep up. I said, 'I think I need an epidural.'

Our wonderful midwife, Ali, was our rock that day, and she'll always be an angel in my eyes. She and I have gone on to become good friends – how can you begin to thank someone enough for delivering the most precious thing to you into the world?

The pushing stage lasted an hour and forty-five minutes,

which was really long, although to me it felt like five minutes. I could feel Lola moving down each time I pushed, then back a bit each time I stopped. Eventually, Ali said, 'We're going to have to get the consultant in. The baby needs to come out, now.' With that, I pushed with all my might for the final time, and Lola was born.

Harry and I were in floods of tears. I asked him to tell me whether our baby was a boy or a girl, then I caught sight of the umbilical cord and thought she was a boy. 'No, she's a girl!' Harry cried. 'She's a girl!' You can't describe the moment when you meet your baby for the first time, something you've dreamed about for ever. All of a sudden there they are, in your arms, more precious than anything. We were euphoric.

Moments after Lola was born, echoing something he'd once said when I was at my very lowest and believed I would never have a child, Harry said to me, 'Izzy, worst case scenario, it's the three of us.'

I couldn't believe it. I'd been lucky enough to see Lola as an embryo, I'd seen the flash of light on the monitor as she was put back home all those months earlier, and finally, after nine months, here she was. I know Harry and I will never forget that moment. For a very long time I'd thought this day would never arrive, and that I would never hold my own baby. The weeks, days and hours I had spent miserable and in the darkest places I have ever been suddenly vanished. She was here and every second of the pain and heartache had been worth the wait. I remember looking at Lola just minutes old and thinking, 'I would wait for ever for you.'

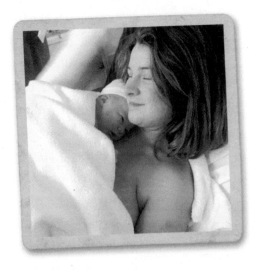

That first night of Lola's life was so surreal and so wonderful. It was just the three of us, together in our hospital room. Harry was asleep, I was wide awake, and Lola was there beside us, in a clear plastic cot. I felt so sorry for her, lying there in the big, wide world on her own, and I missed her. I began to really feel how separated we were from each other now. All I wanted to do was hold her, but I worried I'd fall asleep and she'd fall. I missed her being inside me and it upset me to think she might be feeling lonely too, that perhaps she missed being inside me and felt odd in her clothes, in a cot, on her own. She slept peacefully but eventually, by 4 a.m., I couldn't wait any longer for her to wake and need me for the next feed, I just had to hold her. So for the rest of the night she slept on my chest. It's the closest to heaven I've ever been.

14

Lola and me

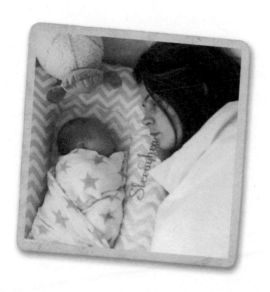

WHEN YOU GO through IVF – at least, this is how it was for me – your investment is in getting pregnant and staying pregnant, and delivering a baby safely. When that's all you've wanted, you don't think so much about the next bit. I'd certainly never really thought about how I'd actually manage with a tiny baby.

Walking out of hospital with Lola the day after she was born, I thought, 'What now?' I now know that, like so many women, I was totally underprepared for becoming a mother.

I hadn't given a moment's real thought to how life was going to change. I'd thought about how many white babygros I needed, and which bath and buggy I'd get, but these are all just ways of giving the illusion that you're in control. As if the right buggy will protect you from the chaos that's about to hit your life! It doesn't matter how many books you read or how many people tell you how different your life will be. Until it happens, you cannot truly imagine the reality.

When we arrived home the first evening with Lola, I had such a funny mix of emotions. Obviously there was the total elation of finally having her home and her being in the world safely, but I also had a weird feeling of real grief for Harry and me, that it was never going to be just us two again. I looked at him holding Lola and thought, 'This is now different for ever,' and I suddenly felt very sad. The last two and a half years of our lives had been so focused on having a baby – we'd been so caught up in it – that when I looked at him, I felt as if it was the first time I'd seen him properly in all that time. It was only now it was no longer just us that I fully realized what we'd lost, even though we'd gained so much.

Before Lola, all of my energies had been ploughed into Harry. We'd had all those years of it being just the two of us, and we'd been through so much together. I loved being a wife, and being at home to take care of him, but now I had a new baby and it's impossible to split yourself – you have to make a choice.

The moment of giving birth is so intense and somehow you have to come down from that. I guess the drop in hormones and adrenaline brings you back to earth with a bang. Certainly that's how I felt in the first few days after having Lola. In fact, my hormones were far crazier in those early days and weeks than they'd been at any time during the process of conceiving or being pregnant. And for that I'd like to make an official apology to Harry!

I began to learn that there are many complicated emotions following birth. Nothing prepared me for the guilt I felt at finding those first weeks hard. When I was trying to fall pregnant I'd spent so long looking at mums with their babies and thinking, 'How lucky you are.' Now that I was one of the lucky ones, I found that nothing was the way I'd expected it to be.

I couldn't get over the overwhelming feeling of responsibility – I didn't know what had hit me. I felt so sorry for Lola because she couldn't tell me what she wanted, and I was deeply unsure what her cries meant. When she was first born, I'd reach for Google every time she started to cry, to try to figure out what was wrong with her. But then I'd say to myself, 'Wait a minute, slow down. What does your instinct say?' I had to learn to trust myself, and that was difficult.

I found breastfeeding very hard at first. I'd left hospital within twenty-four hours of giving birth, having done one latch, and I was very soon at the point of giving up. I didn't find it physically easy at all – in fact, breastfeeding was far more of a challenge for me than labour had been. Lola had difficulty latching on to one side, so I couldn't feed her from there and was expressing instead.

The day my milk came in was pure chaos. My breasts were so engorged. There seemed to be milk flying all over the place and plates of cabbage leaves were scattered everywhere, because I'd heard they could help with the pain of engorgement. There was the noise of the breast pump whirring as I tried to express, and plenty of tears, mine mostly. I was in pain from the birth, exhausted and miserable. Harry was hand expressing for me – we were trying anything we could to get Lola fed – and nothing was as I'd imagined. I felt real guilt then that I wasn't in this blissful bubble. I'd wanted this for so long, and there I was, upset and in shock.

When Lola was five days old we rang a lactation consultant, Clare Byam-Cook, in desperation. Harry left a message for her and she called back immediately, saying, 'I know that when the husband rings, it's urgent!' She arrived at our house within forty-five minutes, and it was as if God had walked in. She took in the scene of chaos and began to create order.

The first thing to do was get Lola fed and settled, so we gave her a bottle and she went to sleep. Clare set to expressing my milk, and thank goodness for breast pumps – I can't tell you the relief I felt having been so engorged! Clare then showed me how to position myself comfortably to breastfeed, talked me through how to get Lola to latch on without pain, and answered all my concerns. Her voice was calm, comforting and reassuring. When Lola woke, Clare got me nursing her from both sides painlessly. The community midwife had suggested that Lola might be tongue-tied and possibly in need of an operation, and I was worried that she might not be able to breastfeed successfully.

Lola does have a slight tongue-tie but she was able to feed perfectly well, so we pretty quickly decided not to have the operation done. We got a second opinion from our doctor, who felt the tongue-tie wasn't serious.

Harry did everything he could to support me during those early weeks of breastfeeding – he made sure I always had water next to me and would feed me healthy food throughout the day to keep my energy levels up. He would even put a snack by my bed for when I'd get up for the night feeds and changes – but there was only so much he could do while I was still breastfeeding.

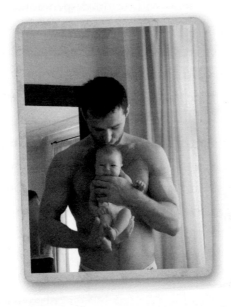

We agreed from the start that I'd do the nights, because of Harry's job and the fact that he really suffers from lack of sleep. He could have changed nappies, I suppose, but because I was awake anyway I decided that I might as well do everything. That way he could get a good night's sleep and be ready to help in the morning while I went back to bed for a few hours.

That was how we worked it out – there was no point

in us both being exhausted – and I was happy with it as an arrangement. I used to lean over and slip his eye mask on and ear plugs in when I was doing night feeds, so that the light and noise wouldn't wake him. And I must have done a good job because many mornings he'd wake up and go, 'Oh, that was a good night last night,' even though I might have been up six times! And yes, there were occasions during the night when I'd look at him with something like hatred, as he lay sound asleep while I was up and feeding! But he more than made up for it because he was amazing during the day and I was able to get plenty of rest.

From the very start, Harry has been a wonderful dad, and is wonderful to me too. He's brilliant with Lola and so happy to do everything for her. She's his world. I can see that she'll be Daddy's little girl for ever, and will get round him effortlessly. It's such a pleasure to watch them together. And that's changed our relationship, too – in a good way.

The first six weeks post-birth are, I believe, difficult for nearly every new mother. You're tired, uncomfortable and uncertain. But I wonder, when you've been through years of trying, and longing desperately for a baby, does that make it even more difficult? Is the pressure to be happy maybe that bit more intense and, if so, are the guilt and confusion at also feeling exhausted and tearful, more intense too? I don't know if it's the same for every mum who's been through IVF to have their baby, but I do know that's how I felt.

Lola was such a good baby and a great sleeper from the start. I'd often look at her and she'd be absolutely fine, snoozing peacefully – it was me who was in a state, awake at all hours and overwhelmed by it all. Lola and I were like the two parts of the metaphorical duck: I was the one furiously pedalling underwater while Lola was floating serenely on the surface.

The body temperature thing stressed me out the most. It's drummed into you (rightly so) about babies overheating, and I'd wonder constantly, 'Is she too hot? Is she too cold?' In the beginning, I took her temperature all the time, touching her forehead, hands and tummy. I'm less anxious about it now, but it can still keep me awake sometimes, especially if she's poorly. It drives Harry mad!

Even after Clare's help, I wasn't the kind of mum who could breastfeed easily when out and about, or wherever we happened to be – I needed to be at home, topless, with five pillows and plenty of space around us. We needed peace and quiet because we were both still learning the business of how to do it. It could take us a few goes to get the latch correct, and doing that in public was something I could never achieve discreetly or without milk spurting everywhere!

Looking back, I wish I hadn't bothered trying to leave the house so much during the early days; that I hadn't put pressure on myself to get out, and had just been happy to sit indoors for however long it took to get a feeding routine sorted. Every time I did go out, I was so tense that my shoulders would be up as high as my ears. Once I'd fed Lola, I knew I had about a three-hour window until she'd be hungry again, so would set about getting ready to go out immediately. But by the time you've changed your clothes and the baby, and packed everything you need in the changing bag, there seems to be barely any time left. Plus, Lola was never very happy in her pram in those early days. I could put her down in her SnuzPod fine if she was swaddled, but in the pram there was too much room and too many sudden bumps, and she just cried and cried. Once I'd discovered babywearing when she was a few weeks old, we got along much better. I adored having her in the sling; to have Lola close again was my favourite thing.

As well as it taking an age to get out of the house, when we were finally out and about I'd become consumed with panic that she'd need a feed before we were able to get home again – and if I didn't make it in time, she'd start crying, and then I'd start crying. I'd see other mums from my NCT class, and they always seemed to be doing so much better. I don't know if they actually were, but that's what it looked like.

I quickly discovered that once you have a baby, your time is not your own, and your mind is not your own. You can't walk away. It's as if the umbilical cord still connects you. If Harry and I ever did go out, I couldn't relax at all, my thoughts would be consumed by Lola and what she might need. And every time I thought I'd nailed it, that I knew what I was doing, Lola would move on to a new phase. I was constantly playing catch-up, and she was always one step ahead of me.

We were fortunate in that we had support. Both our mums were amazing. Harry's mum cooked us loads of meals for the freezer – the best gift anyone can give a new family is healthy, home-cooked, nutritious food. (And

Harry and I soon discovered there was no point cooking food for both of us at once – we had to have two sittings and take it in turns to eat!) Another wonderful gift was that my mum would take all our laundry away with her when she visited and bring it back the next day, beautifully clean and ironed.

When Rupert first visited, he immediately gave me a big hug and asked, 'Are you OK? Was it painful? I was really worried about you.' I remember thinking that he was the only person who wanted to hold me first, not Lola, and ask how I was. That sums up just how loving and caring his nature is. And of course, we all had a chuckle about him asking if childbirth was painful.

I remember the moment Rupert picked up Lola for the first time. I was amazed at just how gentle he was with her. He held her like he'd been holding babies all his life. He kissed her nose gently before putting her back down carefully, then asked if we could all go to the pub!

But despite the love and support, I wish we hadn't had so many other visitors quite so soon. Harry got really excited and wanted people to come and see us, and of course our families and friends all wanted to visit because they were so eager to meet Lola (and that really was lovely). Meanwhile, I was just in a fog. I didn't know what time it was or what was happening, and there were days when I didn't feel like I'd held Lola at all because she was being passed around so many different people.

I think I did get the baby blues. I definitely felt low. Within the first week, a health visitor came to the house and did a questionnaire with me – the routine type they always do about how you're feeling. Are you tearful? Irrational? Overwhelmed? I answered everything honestly and she said I was borderline in terms of mood so she'd come back and check on me in six weeks. By the time she did, I was absolutely fine and much happier. It was the very early days that I found so difficult.

That phase doesn't last for ever, though, despite it feeling like it might – you think you'll never do anything for the rest of your life except sit on the sofa and feed your baby. But it passes, like everything else.

Now, I miss those early days, especially the night feeds. I used to put my little light on and sit there, nursing Lola while looking out the window, wondering which other mums were also up feeding at that time. There was something so lovely about it, in the dark and quiet.

In fact, every time a stage in her development finishes, I feel so much sadness, even though I might have been willing her on to reach the next milestone. Once the new stage comes, I miss the little things she doesn't do any more. Like the first time she sat up beautifully on her own and didn't need me to support her, or when she slept in her own room for the first time – I felt so lonely without her. The last time I breastfed her was the toughest – she just stopped wanting the breast as she loved her bottle too much. At least she was happy, and that's all that really matters.

Harry and I always said we wouldn't be 'that couple' who obsess over their child and talk about nothing else. Well, we are that couple! Maybe when you're looking after a little one there's no other way to be? You're in such a little bubble that sometimes you have no perspective. There are days when I'll ring my mum, we'll talk for an hour about Lola and only at the end will I ask, 'How are you?' There's just no space for anyone or anything except your baby when they're tiny.

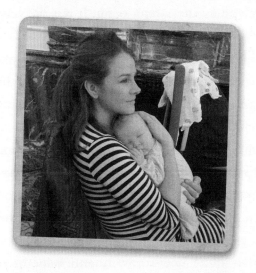

It seems almost funny to say it, but one of the biggest things I had to learn after Lola was born was that she's not me. She's her own little person, with her own personality. She's taught me this herself, as I watch the way she goes about things and responds. I don't think she has the kind of worrying nature I have. In fact, I get the feeling that she's my opposite, and before long will probably start telling me, 'Come on, Mum, pull yourself together!'

At night, when I put her down, she's in a blacked-out room with no lights on anywhere, and I think, 'I'd be so terrified!' But she's perfectly happy. Give her a bunny and she's absolutely fine. I've got a sense that she's a determined little thing – she knows what she wants, just like her daddy!

Something that fascinated me early on with Lola was watching her breathing – babies know how to breathe properly from their tummies. Seeing Lola's belly rise and fall peacefully as she sleeps reminds me how we should breathe naturally. It's something we all knew how to do instinctively when we were tiny, back before life got in the way and tension meant we started breathing from our chests. Watching Lola breathing is one of the most peaceful things. Long, deep breaths from the tummy help soothe anxiety.

It reminds me that we have taught ourselves fear. I don't believe it's innate – everything we dread and worry about is something we've learned. Babies don't use up their energy worrying and thinking about the future, their whole attention is in the moment. They don't experience fear because they don't know how to anticipate; there is such beauty and naivety in that.

I've also learned that I can't control what Lola wants. The way I managed my life before she was born was to control everything that I could. I'd map things out, plan ahead, know exactly what was happening and when. That's how I liked to function. But with Lola, right from the start that wasn't possible. I had to learn a new way of living, and I have done. Which makes me think, perhaps you're sent what you need.

When Harry and I were first thinking about having a family, I worried whether I'd be able to be a good mum because of my anxiety. Could I care for a child in the way it needed? And yet, ironically, since having Lola I haven't had a single anxiety attack. That's not to say I don't have anxieties around her, say, if she's not well or hasn't eaten much one day, all the usual things. But they're around her, not me. I've had moments in the evening after Lola's gone to bed when I've felt tense, but so far I've always been able to say to myself, 'Lola's upstairs, Izzy, pull yourself together.' And that's worked, along with a bit of conscious breathing and some distraction techniques.

When you suffer with anxiety, you're constantly operating in the past or the future, very rarely in the here and now. With a baby, you can only be present and in the moment with them, and I'm sure that's why I'm coping better. Anxiety will always be there but it definitely feels different now. More manageable.

I believe there's always a reason why we experience the things we do. And for me, my fertility struggles, going through IVF and becoming a mum have given me a deeper understanding of who I am and my anxiety. I've learned that you can't control everything and the sooner you can let go the easier life becomes.

15

Amazing things will happen

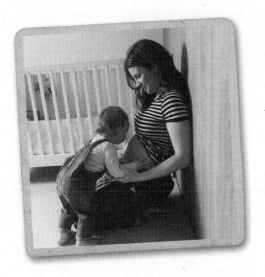

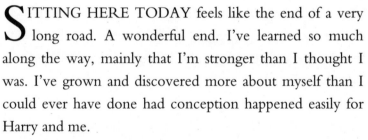

SITTING HERE TODAY feels like the end of a very long road. A wonderful end. I've learned so much along the way, mainly that I'm stronger than I thought I was. I've grown and discovered more about myself than I could ever have done had conception happened easily for Harry and me.

Lola is one year old now, and she's always doing something new and amazing. Doing things with her, noticing her discover things for the first time, seeing her begin to form relationships with other loved ones, and watching her and Harry together is endlessly fascinating and beautiful. There really is something about children – they bring new life and magic to a family, just as I always believed. So, yes, being a mum is everything I ever hoped and wished it would be.

When the time comes to talk to Lola about periods and

fertility, I want to teach her not just about taking precautions but also about her reproductive health. I'll make sure she understands what actually happens when she starts her periods – what's normal and what's not normal. Most of us don't have any real idea what goes on during our cycles, even though it's something that happens to us every month and is such a large and important part of our physical make-up.

And I'll tell her the story of her conception, too – I've never considered not being open about what it took for us to have her. I always felt it was really important to be honest with Lola about what we went through.

Although *Hello!* had featured our wedding and engagement, when they wanted to cover our pregnancy announcement we briefly considered saying no. I felt the only way I could do the interview was if I was completely honest about everything we'd experienced, and that would mean opening up fully. The thought of that scared me initially. How would I feel once the words were out there, written down in black and white for anyone to read? Then I thought, 'Why should we miss out on the opportunity to talk about our experience and share the happy news of our pregnancy?' I'm so pleased we did.

It would have felt dishonest not to talk about how Lola had been conceived. I couldn't have posed for photographs and spoken to the journalists while keeping hidden what we'd been through to get to that happy point, because I knew exactly how other people's pregnancy announcements had made me feel. I wanted to be nothing but open about our struggle.

I felt that IVF and miscarriage were two very important subjects to talk about as they are so much more common than people realize. If we hadn't been as honest as we were, I'd have felt like we were almost ashamed of our IVF journey. And I wasn't ashamed at all. Also, I don't like holding things in. It makes me uncomfortable. I'd rather just come out and tell the truth. I understand that IVF is a deeply personal experience, and I would never have wanted to talk publicly about it while we were going through it – at that stage, it felt completely private – but once I was pregnant and everything was going well, I could see no reason not to.

I don't judge anyone who chooses not to speak about fertility problems because that's their choice. But I felt as if I had a duty to respect other couples who were struggling. I knew how much I'd have appreciated reading about somebody who had gone through what I was going through, and seeing that person with a happy outcome.

Nothing could have prepared me for the warmth I received from those around me and also from total strangers. I got the most amazing response from couples across the country, who got in touch to say that they had been or were in a similar position, and how much of a difference it had made to them to read about someone discussing IVF as something normal, not something shameful to be hidden.

The words 'hope', 'honest' and 'positive' were the ones I probably came across most frequently in the many responses I got. The women were worried, and sometimes confused and scared. Many were finding that they couldn't talk to their friends, because they just didn't understand.

They were desperate for information, for stories, and for advice about how best to prepare themselves, physically and psychologically, for the IVF process to give themselves the very best chance of conceiving.

I recognized that place they were finding themselves in, and it's a very lonely, depressing and uncertain one. You feel frightened and out of control, full of uncertainty about the future, and you can suffer from a lack of confidence and self-belief. It can be as if you're completely losing sight of who you are. You distance yourself from the people around you because you think they can't possibly understand, and you try to walk the path alone. This knowledge and understanding is why I decided to write this book and tell my story fully. That, and the wish to share things I learned along the way that I think could be helpful.

Behind that clinical term, IVF, there are so many stories. Some are very sad, some have wonderful happy endings, but the narrative around those three letters is mostly negative: it's always about the toll it takes on your body, the intrusion and indignity of it, the chances of success which vary hugely from person to person. For me, like so many other things in life, it comes down to how you choose to look at it. I made a decision to be as positive as I could be. Don't get me wrong, that's a very easy thing to say but takes work to do. It's also very difficult to get things back on track if you have a setback, but I truly believe the mind is an amazing and very powerful thing.

I've always felt, any time I've been through anything really big, that I want to do something with that experience, and to try to help other people. I've learned that from my mum and it was one of the reasons I set up the Eyes Alight appeal, to support people like Rupert who have suffered brain injuries. And so, knowing what I now know about IVF, I'd like to encourage more openness around the subject and create a community where people can come together to share experiences, talk to other women who find themselves in similar situations, and share stories of hope.

People often ask me if I'm a more overprotective mother to Lola because of the way in which she was conceived. I think the answer is that I would be the same mother whatever had happened. I don't believe having gone through IVF makes me any different; I'd be just as worried about Lola, would love her just as much, however she had arrived.

Every baby is delicate and a miracle. IVF is how we conceived Lola, but now that she's here I'd never like her to think she's more special, more precious, than any other child.

For a while I thought, what next? I grew up wanting a big family, because I come from one. I know that Harry and I are blessed to have Lola, and if she's all that we are given I would be content with that. But I also know I'd love for her to have a sibling.

One of the truly wonderful things that happened during the course of writing this book is that I found out I was pregnant. It all happened naturally and so our next little miracle has been a beautiful surprise.

Almost as soon as Lola was born, people – usually the same

ones who used to say, 'Just relax and it'll happen' – began telling me, 'Oh, you'll probably fall pregnant naturally next time' and 'You often hear about people falling pregnant naturally after having IVF.' I know it was meant with kindness but it frustrated me because I really didn't believe them. I wondered how would it ever be that simple after all the difficulties we had previously faced. I thought, 'As if I would ever be so lucky.'

Harry and I always said, 'Why would we ever not try? After everything we've been through, if another pregnancy were to happen naturally, it would be amazing.' So we never took precautions after Lola was born, and when my cycle came back, as it did eight months after her birth, I felt so excited. The first time I got my period, I ran down the stairs, shouting, 'Harry, you'll never guess what!' at the top of my voice. I was so proud of my body!

I still didn't believe I would conceive naturally, though. Harry and I had already begun to talk about what we might do next and the kind of age gap we might like between Lola and her sibling, if we were ever lucky enough to have another child. However, I didn't feel ready for another round of IVF. I'd spent so long waiting for Lola that I wanted to enjoy our time together – I didn't want the early years with her to be consumed by medical appointments. But I also grew worried about leaving it too long. Even though we still have one frozen embryo, I got to the point where I considered freezing more eggs while I was still in my early thirties.

We hadn't made any decisions but in the background part of me was thinking, 'What if I am one of those women who gets pregnant after IVF?' At the same time, another part was thinking, 'That won't be you!' Even now, I can't help wondering, 'How can it suddenly be so easy, when it was so hard before?' It's something I still find very difficult to get my head around.

Once pregnancy was even a faint possibility, then of course I became highly aware of my body again, and how I was feeling at different points during the month. I wanted to find out whether I was ovulating or not, so I decided to track my cycle to see what was going on.

In December 2016, I tested from Day Eleven for six days with a home ovulation kit – more peeing on sticks – because that's the time during which an egg would usually be released in a twenty-eight-day cycle. Each day the result was negative. I wasn't ovulating. I presumed then that things were just back to how they were before – I'd get my period but without having ovulated.

Despite the discouraging results, I still did a pregnancy test on Day Twenty-eight of my cycle. I'd had a really bad stitch in my side a few days before and had been wondering, 'What's that?' I confess that I even googled 'stitch in early pregnancy', just in case. Of course this just left me worried when one of the search results suggested it might be a symptom of an ectopic pregnancy. I also felt suspicious when Murphy kept curling up right next to my tummy at night – he's such an intuitive cat. It brought back so many memories of trying to hold on to anything that might be a sign! I was also getting reflux and wanted to eat stodgy food but I thought, 'As if!' It was Christmas, after all.

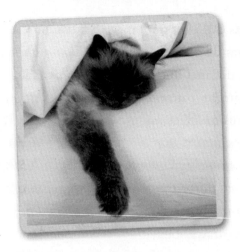

*Murphy, my loyal companion
for so many years.*

Anyway, I did the test on Day Twenty-eight, which happened to be Christmas Day. It was negative, but that was fine. If anything I felt a little silly for even thinking I might be pregnant.

After Christmas my family, Harry and I travelled to Somerset to see my cousins. I noticed I was very hormonal, tearful and grumpy – it felt like I was waiting for my period to start. I don't usually tend to have PMT but this was bad, and I felt really crampy. Three days later, in the evening, I did another test because I still hadn't had my period. It still showed negative.

I was upset, disappointed and worried. I was also afraid I was slipping back into the obsession that had gripped me before, of googling and watching and hoping, and always being disappointed. You'd think I'd have learned from my mistakes! I texted my brother Magnus that day, because he'd asked if I was OK after our visit to the cousins – I think he'd noticed I was distracted. 'My period hasn't started again so I'm feeling deflated about the chances of falling pregnant naturally. Similar patterns forming. I will stay positive, I refuse for this to affect my precious early years with Lola,' my message said.

But back home in London, I began to think, 'My cycle last month was thirty-five days, perhaps I've tested too soon. Maybe I should just do one more …' Part of me felt I was clutching at straws, but another part of me was curious, wondering where my period was.

So on New Year's Eve I bought some cheap supermarket home pregnancy tests and on New Year's Day 2017 I got up, took Lola downstairs with me, went into the loo and tested. And there was a line! I couldn't believe it! 'Look, Lola, there's a line! There's a line!' Bless little Lola, she was just looking up at me, smiling. I rushed up to Harry then, and said, 'Morning, Happy New Year, and look!' Being half asleep it took him a little while to take in what I was actually showing him.

Eventually he said, 'That's definitely a line! That's a good line.' He was wide awake now! It felt like a miracle to us, and the fact that it was New Year's Day made it all the more so.

We told our families immediately because we knew that if anything were to happen, we'd need their support. There was a moment when I was tempted to wait until twelve weeks and surprise them but I suppose that wish to be able to make the dream announcement has been taken away from me. The support from my family is more important and hiding the pregnancy during those early weeks would have put more pressure on me. I'm writing this now for the same reason. Whatever happens next, I want to be open and honest.

We also know that we still have a little embryo sitting in the freezer with a woolly hat on, and that we'll have to make a decision about it at some point. We can't leave it there. To us, it isn't just an embryo. We know what kind of life is there, because we've seen it; we've experienced Lola being born. Luckily, there's no rush to make the decision. In the meantime, I'm determined to take each day as it comes.

Looking at Lola, holding her, having her with me and Harry makes this experience of pregnancy very different. I look at her and think it's thanks to her that I've fallen pregnant naturally. It's almost as if my system was reset after

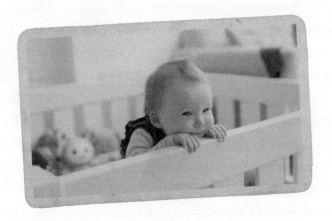

*I feel it's thanks to Lola that I've
fallen pregnant naturally.*

giving birth – and I'm sure Lola made it cosy in there for her brother or sister to settle in comfortably! I still have anxiety around what could happen: I look forward to my scans and feel relief afterwards, and I feel delighted by how sick and tired I feel. But I also know that whatever comes next, we have Lola, and Harry and I have each other.

With both rounds of IVF, I knew precisely where I was from very early on of course, whereas this time, for a while I didn't know exactly how many weeks pregnant I was. So it was fantastic, and such a relief, when I went to the first scan at around seven weeks and found that I'd already passed the six-weeks-and-four-days milestone – the day when I'd had the miscarriage – without having to go through it consciously.

Just like last time, we won't find out if we're having a boy or a girl, because we loved the element of surprise we had with Lola. I think you always feel a degree of caution about how much you allow yourself to dream about having a baby – but if I do allow myself to go there with this pregnancy, I'm incredibly excited at the thought of giving Lola a brother or sister, and of growing our family.

I daydream about how the baby might look – will they resemble Lola or be completely different? I think about holding them for the first time and about Lola meeting them. I adore my brothers and hope Lola and her brother or sister can have the same amazing relationship as we do.

For all that I'm delighted to have fallen pregnant naturally this time, I'll always feel Lola was conceived just the way she was supposed to be. She's taught me so much and now

Number 2 is already teaching me a totally new set of lessons. I'm sure the learning curve will continue with both of them.

I do believe that everything happens for a reason. And yes, I struggle with the reason for Rupert's accident, but then I see the joy he brings and the lessons he's taught me and so many others. I also find the thought of our miscarriage heartbreaking, and I'm not sure I'll ever find peace with our loss. I suppose some stars shine just that little bit brighter – Rupert and our little soul will always be those stars.

We dared to dream.

My side of the story, by Harry

HAVING CHILDREN has always been one of my goals in life. I grew up in a close-knit family – I'm the youngest of three – and strong morals and good manners were ingrained in us by our parents. I was brought up to respect the idea of family, and I always knew that eventually I would want one of my own.

Izzy and I first met in 2005, in a church in Bristol where McFly were rehearsing for our *Wonderland* tour. I noticed Izzy immediately, not just because I thought she was really pretty but because she has a kind face. I walked over to her while my bandmates and I were introducing ourselves to the members of the orchestra, and gave her a kiss on the cheek. 'I'm Harry,' I said, and we smiled at each other.

It wasn't until the end of the tour that we got together as a couple, and I was certain straight away that it was something serious. Our first week together was a whirlwind; intense and exciting. I knew very quickly – within a few weeks – that Izzy was the person I wanted to be with, although I think it took her a little longer to be convinced! I remember clearly the exact moment when I told her how I felt. It was in the kitchen of our band house and I said, 'Izzy, you don't understand, I'm going to marry you one day.' I was only nineteen years old! After that, we were both quick to say 'I love you' – there was no messing around.

Izzy is such a genuine person, and I guess that's what I realized I was looking for. At that age, in the music scene, you end up meeting a lot of people who are into drinking and partying – it can be pretty superficial. I'd joined in for a couple of years but by the time I met Izzy, I was starting to get tired of it. Although I'd met some great people along the way, I hadn't felt a proper connection with anyone for ages, so I was ready for a real relationship. And with Izzy, it just felt right.

In general, there's a really good balance in our relationship. Neither of us wears the trousers – we share that role. It's important to have that kind of equality – if one person dominates, it can squash the other. A friend of mine once said of me and Izzy, 'You both need each other as much as the other', which is to say we both have vulnerability and strength.

The only thing that's ever caused any real friction in our relationship is Izzy's anxiety, but we found a way, together, to live with it, and we overcame the challenges it presented. Maybe having had to deal with those earlier difficulties helped when we came up against the challenges of fertility, because we'd already been through a lot together. We'd learned patience and kindness.

Our fertility struggles changed the dynamic between us, too. Previously, I'd been the one who was busy with the band and doing lots of other things, and Izzy was the one propping me up. Once we started IVF, though, I became a support to Izzy. It was my turn to be the one who was patient and calm.

When Izzy first missed her period, we were both certain that it was good news. We were in our old house at the time, and Izzy told me that she'd been feeling a bit odd – she'd been googling early signs of pregnancy because she thought she might be pregnant. I remember feeling so excited and emotional, and thinking about how amazing it was that we were going to be parents. How totally naive that seems now.

When we visited my parents around that time, I had a long chat with my mum about kids. I almost told her that Izzy was pregnant, even though Izzy hadn't taken the test yet. Izzy just looked so well – she was glowing, plus her cycle had always been like clockwork and she'd now missed her period. There couldn't be any other explanation.

The day we did the pregnancy test, we were so sure it was going to be positive that I was ready to capture the moment with my camera. I was convinced that it would be something we would show our child on their twenty-first birthday or some equally significant celebration. So when the test was negative, we were both really confused.

Izzy always maintained that she wasn't going to be one

of those women who obsesses over ovulation and pees on sticks, that she'd be really chilled about the whole thing. I was happy too to just go with the flow and be relaxed, whether it took six months or even a year. Instead, what happened? Izzy peed on the stick, got a negative result and immediately – panic. Call the doctor. We went from nought to one hundred instantly, and stayed at one hundred.

Although I wanted Izzy to calm down, I understood her concern. Why had her period not come when it had always been so regular? She's an anxious person, so I knew she needed to find out – and that was the start of it. Sometimes I look back and think, 'If only we'd just fallen pregnant that first month, and had never known any of this – the ups and downs, the endless trips and scans and doctor's appointments. The tears, anxiety, feeling low, the disappointment …'

As the months passed and Izzy took all the medication she did, and went for endless scans, I felt my role was to support her. But I also wanted to try to take her mind off everything that was happening, to give her a different focus if possible. I tried to give rational advice and if I could see that she was trying to justify leaping into more interventions, I'd encourage her to try to look at things more objectively.

At the time, Izzy had just left her profession – from the age of four, she'd trained to be a violinist, and now she'd stepped away from it. She'd set up her own business, Izzy's Attic, but her mind wasn't really on that as she was so focused on wanting to start a family. Because of this, there was an urgency in her that I'd never seen before – she wanted to do whatever it took to get pregnant. When it didn't happen, she'd ask why and what could she do to fix it, be it injections, pills, whatever. We tried all kinds of different things but none of them worked. And of course, this all started shortly after our wedding. It should have been a happy time but getting pregnant completely took over her whole existence.

The medication Izzy took affected her both emotionally and physically. She totally lost her confidence and her dynamism, and she didn't feel like herself. Nothing I could do or say helped. If I was invited to a party, she no longer wanted to come with me and if she did come, she didn't really want to be there. She'd travel with us on tour because she didn't want to be at home on her own, but in reality there was a large part of her that just wanted to hide away. She'd sit at the front of the tour bus, away from all the guys, hidden away under a hoodie, and I realized that everyone must be wondering what was up with her. It was hard but I always really tried to keep her spirits up.

As time went on there was frustration on both our parts. Izzy was angry that she'd been taking the fertility drugs for months and months and they didn't seem to be having any effect – she still wasn't ovulating. She resented the fact that she was pumping herself full of stuff that just wasn't doing anything for her. Of course, I felt sorry for how she was feeling, but I was frustrated too because I just wanted her to be happy – and I also really wanted my old Izzy back. I'd even sometimes say to close friends, 'We haven't even had a baby yet and already I'm over it.' To me, it didn't matter whether we had a baby right then or in a few years' time, but because I wanted to support Izzy I didn't share those feelings with her.

After a pretty miserable year, Izzy decided to stop all medical intervention. Instead, she embarked on a mission to be super healthy, and that's when I saw a real change in her. It was amazing. She went from being miserable, low, depressed and feeling sorry for herself to having a completely different attitude. She found the strength of character to pick herself up, and got going with incredible focus and determination. She ate like a goddess, exercised and meditated to get her mind in check.

Even though she was amazing in her ability to stick to her plan, doing all these things to be healthy and calm and positive, we still didn't get the result we wanted – a positive pregnancy test never materialized. That's when we began to talk about IVF seriously. Izzy really wanted to do it but I was unsure at first. I didn't feel there was any hurry to rush into more fertility treatment, and the headspace Izzy had been in since her detox was such a good one that I didn't want her to risk slipping back into a dark place. The truth is, I worried that if IVF didn't work, we'd have nowhere else to turn, and I couldn't bear the thought of seeing Izzy in that situation.

IVF meant that Izzy had to pump herself with more medication, but she remained positive every step of the way. She kept saying, 'This will happen. We will get there in the end.' Every time she injected herself with the drugs, she'd say, 'This is bringing us one step closer to meeting our baby.' I found her attitude amazing, considering she didn't really know – *couldn't* know – that 'this' would happen. She stuck with it, though, and that part of the experience became an exciting one, when it could easily have been miserable and negative.

So what was my role in the IVF process? First and foremost there was sperm collection and, yes, it's a little bit odd, but I was shown into a room and I just had to get on with it! I was, of course, mindful of how much Izzy was going through. I was so proud of the way she was dealing with it, especially considering she was terrified of lots of things – particularly egg collection because it involved being heavily sedated, and the idea of being out cold made her very anxious. I just felt that we were lucky that science could help us and that I only had to do my part to help.

Once we had a fertilized embryo ready and waiting we went to the transfer, which was incredible. Watching life being placed inside Izzy was amazing. Everybody wonders about the moment a baby is conceived. We were able to see that moment. You'd think it would be really sterile and clinical, but in a way it's romantic. You're there together, you can hold hands. They show you what's happening on a monitor, and that's your moment to just imagine what might be; to have your dream. You look at the screen and think, 'Is that our baby? It's OK if it's not, but there's hope, and we're lucky to have that.'

The night before Izzy was due to take the pregnancy test I rang my mum. I was so nervous that I started crying. It was the first time I'd cried about things but I really wanted the test to be positive, almost for Izzy's sake alone. I felt so sorry for her at this point, as did my mum – we both wanted it so badly for her.

When Izzy did the test and it was positive, I just never believed the result somehow; I never connected with the idea. Maybe I didn't dare? The line on the pregnancy test was really faint, and I know that means nothing – faint or strong, same thing – but I was worried. I couldn't get as excited as Izzy was.

As the days went by, though, I gradually started to let myself believe. It was my birthday, our wedding anniversary and Christmas all in the same week, and I was beginning to feel more positive about things. We allowed ourselves to build up the excitement slowly – we told both our families and I told a couple of my closest mates.

Then, in the early hours of Boxing Day, Izzy woke up and called out to me, saying, 'Harry, Harry, there's blood.' On the inside I was panicking but I had to hide that from her and do everything I could to reassure and support her. Because of the blood, I feared the worst – that she was miscarrying – but Izzy's doctor gave us many explanations as to why this might be happening, so we relaxed a little bit.

A few days later, though, we were driving back to London when Izzy said she wasn't feeling right. She didn't have to say much but I knew that things weren't as they should be. When we got home, I made her soup and toast, and I put the fire and the telly on. Izzy seemed quite calm – we can both be worriers but at no point did either of us actually say, 'Do you think it's a miscarriage?' We never vocalized it, and instead just tried to stay hopeful.

My side of the story, by Harry

The next morning we were due to have our first scan. It was still dark when my alarm went off at 6.30 a.m. I shot out of bed and went downstairs to make Izzy some tea. Then, from the kitchen, I heard her say in a voice filled with adrenaline and panic, 'Harry, we've lost it.' The fact that she said 'it' rather than 'our baby' stayed with me.

'Don't worry, it's OK,' I told her, because I just didn't know what else to say. I was trying to be strong for both of us but we were both in shock and so tired. It was cold and dark, and still so early in the morning that I half wondered if I was dreaming. In a way, I found it hard to be the man in that situation – mine was a secondary loss; I wasn't able to physically connect with it. Izzy, on the other hand, had to cope with the real sensation of the baby passing.

Later that morning we saw our doctor, Ram, who is such a sweet man. He scanned Izzy and I could see on the screen that there was nothing there, just an empty space. We'd spent the previous few weeks talking and thinking about our baby, bringing it to life, asking each other about possible boys' and girls' names. We'd made it real by talking about it, giving it a future. We'd leapt ahead, to the due date, to us as a family, to when the baby was growing up and whether it would look like Izzy or me. Suddenly, all of that was gone. It was devastating. A moment of such emptiness.

I soon found out how common miscarriages are, and I felt stupid for having spent those weeks fantasizing about what would be. I'd got carried away and felt an internal embarrassment at having let my imagination run away with me.

After the scan, Izzy went to the loo. While she was out of the room I asked Ram, 'What do I do with the …?' I didn't even know what to call it – the foetus? The baby? 'It's still there, in the loo. Do I take it out? Do I flush it?' I really didn't know. I didn't want Izzy to have to deal with it. I realized that I had to face it, that this was my job.

Ram was great. 'You can take it out, if you want,' he said. 'Some people like to bury it in the garden. Other people like to flush. There is no right answer – it's up to you and how you feel.'

So I was left with two options. Do I make a thing of this? Do I physically take it out of the loo – in paper, in a plastic bag? Are we ready to go through a burial? To have a funeral, on the day, and forever look at that corner of the garden and know what's there? Or do I do something that seems horribly nonchalant and flush the loo? Is that too disrespectful to that soul?

I couldn't ask Izzy. I knew I had to take responsibility and make a decision. As soon as we got home, I went straight upstairs. I didn't even look, I just flushed the loo and came back down. It was my decision and I thought, 'I'm not going to be either symbolic or cynical about this. I'm just going to do what I feel is right, at this time.'

Izzy was sweet and kept asking me if I was OK. I called my parents and spoke to my mum. You know when you hear your mother's voice, how emotional that can make you feel? Especially when you've been trying to be strong and brave and hold yourself together? She knew we'd had the scan that morning, and as soon as I said, 'Hi, Mum,' she could tell instantly that something was wrong. She asked if everything was OK and I told her the news. I could hear that she was trying to be strong for me, just as I was trying to be strong for Izzy.

I could hear my dad in the background and my mum passed the phone to him. When he heard what had happened, he broke down in tears. It was only the third time I had ever heard my dad cry. The first time was when I was eight years old and I was about to go off to boarding school. My brother was crying, I was crying, my mum was crying. Then my dad started crying and I thought he was joking, teasing us, trying to make us feel better. I started laughing and said, 'Dad, shut up,' before realizing that his tears were for real.

The only other time was when he came to watch me doing *Strictly*. It was Week Nine and we'd done a quickstep, and won the Swingathon. The next morning when I rang my parents, Dad said, 'That was the most fantastic night, last night. You were just brilliant,' and started to cry. That was the first time I'd known him to shed a tear in eighteen years.

That morning after the miscarriage, he and I sobbed on the phone to each other. I really let it out and I think that was a good thing. I felt like all I wanted to do was cry, and so I did. It only happened once more, when we were at the airport on our way to Antigua. Izzy had a headache, and before the plane took off I said she should take some painkillers. She looked at the instructions on the back of the packet. 'Do not take if pregnant,' she read aloud, and we just looked at each other and broke down.

Dare to dream

After the scan, I had to keep myself busy so I spent the afternoon gardening. I was up on the roof, sweeping leaves, cleaning gutters. That's how I tried to cope with the sadness of what had happened. All Izzy wanted was to be pregnant, and she had finally had those few weeks to feel what it was like to carry life inside her. She'd been able to believe that all the horrible things she'd been through were over, and that we just might be allowed to get on with our lives and be a family. But then it had all been snatched away from her. It was a testing time for both of us – we were upset, angry and worried. We knew that we'd have to go through the whole process again and were now painfully aware of everything that could entail.

Within a week or so, I switched into thinking practically whereas Izzy needed a bit more time to process what had happened. I became focused on what we were going to do next, how we were going to move on. I realized that you can't dwell too much on what might have been, and came to understand that miscarriage was nature's way of saying 'not this time'.

The second time Izzy got pregnant, we told our families and friends straight away, so that they could support us, if we needed them to. I didn't want us to be scared and on tenterhooks all on our own.

Everything felt different that second time. I remember being at the transfer and thinking that the embryo looked like a girl, which seems silly, but it was nice for us to have those conversations. 'Good luck, little one,' I said, as we watched the transfer on screen.

My side of the story, by Harry

When it was time to go back to the clinic a week later, to do the blood test to find out if the embryo had successfully implanted, we were unbearably nervous. We were told we'd have to wait thirty minutes for the results, so Izzy suggested we go for a walk to pass the time. We were outside for what felt like half an hour, then went back into the clinic only to find we'd been gone for just five minutes! The nurse called us in finally, and told us that we had a positive result. I couldn't quite believe it so I had to ask her again.

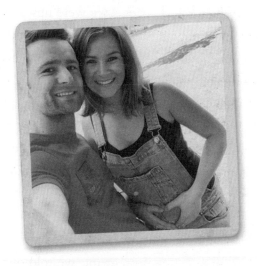

This was the photo we used to go public with our happy news. I was over the moon to see Izzy so happy.

Even when the good news was confirmed, we told ourselves that it was only step one and that it was too early to celebrate. We were cautious, only thinking ahead to the next milestone, the first scan. Something felt better this time around, though. I began counting down the days, the hours, the minutes and seconds, and hoped that getting to the magical twelve-week mark would eliminate the worry. It didn't, not fully, but it helped. The nerves settled a little bit, but it wasn't until we got to about thirty weeks that I started to feel more confident that everything would be OK. It was then that I finally allowed myself to relax more. It was the longest nine months of my life – I was so excited, and so impatient.

I was over the moon at Izzy's joy as the pregnancy progressed. She'd fantasized about walking around with a bump for such a long time. She'd been locked out of that world – seeing pregnant women everywhere she looked, baby shops, people pushing buggies. To see her bump growing and her buying maternity clothes, to hear her talk about the nursery – it was wonderful.

When the time came and Izzy went into labour, I felt really excited. It lasted a long time, but Izzy was remarkable and seemed to know exactly what to do. Some guys talk about their partner giving birth and say stuff like, 'It's like watching your favourite pub burn down.' I think that's such bullshit. Watching Izzy give birth was an incredible and beautiful thing.

When Lola was finally born, Izzy and I were both in floods of tears with the wonder of it all. Izzy thought Lola was a boy at first because she saw the umbilical cord. I'd always thought I wanted to have a boy but when Izzy was nine months pregnant we visited some friends who have a little girl, and she was just the sweetest thing. At that point I began to think it would be quite nice to have a daughter. And then, there she was – our girl.

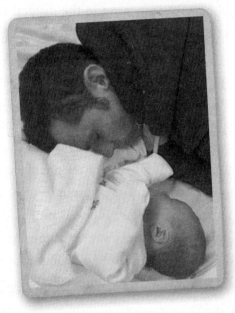

When I saw Lola for the first time, I was on cloud nine – it was a euphoric moment. Some people say that it's the best moment of your life, while others say they didn't really bond with the baby for a few months, so you wonder how you'll react. I was so lucky. From the moment I saw Lola, I was hit with the full whack of love.

When she cries now, it takes me right back to the moment she first cried when I held her as a tiny newborn. I can visualize her first moments as clear as day. Izzy's quite envious because she can't really remember any of it, she was so tired. As I also cried, my tears of joy, I told Lola not to worry, that we would always look after her.

I feel love for Lola like I've never felt. I worry, too, because I absolutely worship her. In a way I'm grateful for what Izzy and I went through to have her – maybe it was a blessing in disguise. Could it have been this good if all those things hadn't happened? I'm not saying that those who conceive easily don't appreciate their children, but there is, to me, something very special about how long we waited.

I wanted Izzy to tell this story because she's at her best when she's helping others. While she's a brilliant musician and performer, she is most fully herself when she's caring for someone else – a husband, a baby, her brother Rupert. I encouraged her to write this book, to share what she's been through and what she's learned along the way, because I knew she'd want to help others by doing so.

When she first spoke openly about having had IVF, the number of people – family, school friends, friends of friends, followers on social media – who contacted her to ask how she did it, how she stayed sane throughout, was phenomenal. Izzy would reply to them all, spending hours on the phone or online, telling them what she did and how she managed the different challenges. She never holds back, she gives so much of herself.

Often, those who are about to have IVF have only heard negative things about it. Whereas Izzy, while she admits it's tough, also lets people know that there's another way to look at it, that it can be amazing and magical. She does a great job of shining a positive light on it for others.

It's wonderful for me to see that Izzy has found herself again. She's got her family and she's got her confidence back. Don't get me wrong, there's a dynamic shift in a relationship when a baby arrives, and never in the man's favour, but I don't mind because we share our love for our daughter. In fact, I think sometimes Izzy thinks that Lola gets more cuddles from me than she does. But you have to work together on things – you have to support each other, and some of your old habits have to die, and die fast, because now you have a baby.

I don't think I ever felt I needed support myself during the process, not massively, but if I did, it came from open and honest conversations with Izzy, my mum and close friends. I talked to Tom, my bandmate, and he was able to sympathize and understand. Izzy and I both gained a lot of comfort from talking, and getting a dose of sympathy from close friends and family. How you deal with it all is an individual choice, but I think it's important to have someone you can open up to other than your partner.

If I was to give advice to a man about to embark on a journey such as ours – and I've done this a couple of times now with friends – I'd say that you just have to be very patient and really supportive. It's not going to be easy. Hormones are going to be messed with and it's going to be a very emotional time. Physically, the procedures are invasive, and yes, sex does become something different when you're trying for a baby – more mechanical – but that all goes back to normal afterwards, and the romance returns.

This time in our lives has been a test for our relationship, there's no doubt about it, and there have been a number of definite shifts – when it comes to Lola Izzy's in charge and I'm vice-captain, a supporting role. There's just something about a mother's instinct that means she's the one to naturally take charge.

We'll have more challenges in our lives and in our marriage, I'm sure. During the difficult times you have to remember your vows: 'For better, for worse … in sickness and in health.' Our struggle was one of the worse times, but we just had to get through it. And we did.

Since Izzy has had Lola, and known the fulfilment of being a mother – the only thing she ever wanted – she's back to herself, and better than ever. I'm just as, if not more, attracted to her because of the way she's handled what she went through. I have a whole new level of respect for her and what she's done.

I'm so proud of her, and of our beautiful daughter.

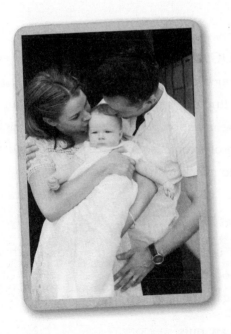

#IzzyLoves

I THOUGHT I'D SHARE with you a few things that I feel helped me during my fertility treatment and IVF. I hope you find my tips useful. Although I spent many hours researching nutrition and supplements, I'm not a qualified medical professional so before making changes to your lifestyle, do check with your doctor.

MY DIET DURING IVF

I avoided caffeine, dairy, gluten and all refined sugars. I chose blood-nourishing foods, and meals that are rich in iron, omega fatty acids and protein, including, for example:

- Mixed raw nuts
- Leafy green vegetables, such as kale and spinach
- Avocados

- Butternut squash
- Aduki bean soup
- Salmon with ginger and spinach
- Mackerel with curly kale
- Steak with cumin-roasted sweet potato
- Beetroot risotto
- Lentil stew
- Warm raw cacao with cinnamon and unsweetened almond milk
- Herbal teas (fennel, nettle and jasmine)
- Plenty of water
- Protein shakes (plant based)

SUPPLEMENTS

For fertility support, I took the following, as directed:

- Magnesium
- Omega 3
- Vitamin D
- Vitamin C
- Probiotic
- Fertility multivitamin

I saw a nutritionist called Alison Belcourt who advised me on which supplements to take: www.alisonbelcourt.co.uk, and I used supplements from the Natural Health Practice: www.naturalhealthpractice.com

#IzzyLoves

BOOKS

Brantley, Jeffrey and Kabat-Zinn, Jon, *Calming Your Anxious Mind* (New Harbinger, 2007)

Byam-Cook, Clare, *What to Expect When You're Breastfeeding … and What If You Can't* (Vermilion, 2006)

Canon, Emma, *Fertile: Nourish and Balance Your Body Ready for Baby Making* (Vermilion, 2017)

Glenville, Marilyn, *Natural Solutions to PCOS* (Macmillan, 2012)

Graves, Katharine, *The Hypnobirthing Book: An Inspirational Guide for a Calm, Confident, Natural Birth* (Katharine Publishing, 2012)

Kite, Gerad, *The Art of Baby-Making: The Holistic Approach to Fertility* (Short Books, 2016)

APPS

Headspace (free sample meditations; in-app purchases required)

Calm (guided meditations to help you sleep and deal with anxiety and stress; in-app purchases required)

GUIDED MEDITATIONS

Zita West
www.zitawest.com/product-category/cds-and-downloads

Maggie Howell
www.natalhypnotherapy.co.uk

HYPNOBIRTHING

Hollie de Cruz

www.londonhypnobirthing.co.uk

I love the London Hypnobirthing Yesmum Fertility and Yesmum To Be Affirmation Cards. There are thirty-one cards in a pack and you can place them somewhere you are likely to see them regularly. I put mine on my bedside table and inside my handbag. They provide a simple daily reminder of a positive thought, which can really help to shift your mindset.

BREASTFEEDING SUPPORT

Clare Byam-Cook

www.clarebyam-cook.com

ACUPUNCTURE

Gerad Kite

www.geradkite.com

#AskIzzy

SINCE OPENING UP about my fertility problems, there are some questions that I'm regularly asked by others experiencing similar struggles. I decided to include an Ask Izzy section here to answer some of those questions, in the hope that my responses will be helpful to anyone going through fertility issues of their own.

How did your fertility problems and IVF journey affect your relationship, and how did you cope with their impact?

The fertility problems that Harry and I experienced, I feel, have brought us closer together. That period of our lives, though, did mark a definite shift in our relationship. Previously, I'd been the steady support to Harry – I was very content with the simple things in life and was happy to be Harry's rock. I think it must have been a big shock for Harry to see me crumble into an insecure and unhappy mess, but his ability to remain patient and his rational mentality helped us both to get through the darkest of days.

At the time, we didn't actually talk about how best to handle our emotions (we were far too busy learning all about my ovaries!) but Harry just seemed to know instinctively what I needed and allowed me to deal with my emotions in my own way. Harry's way of coping when he did have difficult days was to open up to his mum or his close friends – it would've been difficult for him to talk to me about his biggest concerns as they were mostly about me. I often told Harry how responsible and guilty I felt for not being able to get pregnant, but he always eased those worries and made me feel that we were in it together. Looking back, I realize just how much of a rock he was, and I wish I'd appreciated that more at the time.

There's so much waiting … How did you deal with that?

Through all the different stages of our fertility struggles there seemed to be *so* much waiting. During the months I spent on Clomid, I had to wait and see if I'd responded to the medication. Then my periods stopped completely and I endured months and months of waiting for my cycle to come back (it never did). At that point, we decided to go ahead with IVF, but we couldn't start until I'd taken the Pill for nearly a month. When we did finally start IVF, I had to wait and see if I was responding well to the medication. But the longest wait of all was the two-week wait following embryo transfer day – those days felt like months.

Learning to be patient became routine for me. It was quite an education about the pace at which we live our lives today and how we are so used to getting what we want as soon as we want it. It's a skill to learn to slow down and appreciate the moment. I found doing something therapeutic helped me to feel less overwhelmed: a walk in my favourite park, being around nature, finishing off little jobs I had been meaning to do like filling our wedding album, and spending time with loved ones were some of the ways to help with the waiting.

Do anything to make *you* feel happy.

How did you manage the vast range of emotions experienced while undergoing treatment?

At first I didn't manage my emotions well at all: waves of panic surged through me daily. When you start treatment, you're suddenly thrown into a world of uncertainty and the whirlwind of feelings can be overwhelming.

In the early days, I didn't have a single rational thought; I just wanted a baby so badly. As time passed and I began to understand that things weren't going to go as planned (not easy for a control freak to admit!), I started to learn a different way of coping with my emotions and tried my best to learn how to let go. I tried alternative therapies such as acupuncture, yoga and meditation to help me find a sense of calm. I put all of my energy into being the healthiest person I could possibly be, both in body and mind.

Throughout fertility treatment every emotion will hit

you, from guilt and anger to frustration and hope, so it's very important to put yourself first and to surround yourself with the people who are going to love and support you through the best and the worst of you!

What can I do to support a friend going through similar struggles?

I do understand how hard it is to know what to say to someone having difficulties. Despite having been through these struggles myself, I'm still not sure what it is exactly that I'd have wanted someone to say to me! I think the most important thing is to let your friend know that you're there for them. Just a simple 'I'm here if you want to talk about anything', taking the time to understand what they're going through physically and mentally, or even offering practical help – such as giving them a lift to their appointments – means a lot.

My best friend, Chantal, fell pregnant during my struggles, but because she remained so sensitive to my feelings I was able to manage my emotions around it. She also didn't hide anything from me and I didn't hide anything from her. We talked about her pregnancy and we talked about the treatment I was going through.

Everyone is different and copes with their feelings in different ways. Trust that you know your friend or loved one well and that you understand how they tick. Your instinct will be right and the best thing you can do is let them know they have your love and support.

How did you get through the hardest days?

To be honest, I got through the really bad ones by hiding in the house with the cats, wearing my hoodie, crying and watching chick flicks! I suppose you do just get through those days and it helped that Harry was always there to give me a cuddle.

It's important to allow yourself time to be sad, angry, frustrated and lonely – you can't always be positive and proactive. Whenever I had a tough day, I'd usually force myself to get up early the following day and do some exercise. It's amazing how much better that can make you feel, even if it's the last thing you feel like doing.

Was there anything in particular that eased the side effects of the drugs you had to take – or did you just have to get through it?

For me, the side effects of Clomid were the toughest. I became bloated, irritable and I gained weight. I think all that would have been easier to deal with if the drug had worked for me. I know it does work for many women, but the fact that it didn't in my case made me feel very negative. When I started IVF I changed my mindset and began to think of the medications in a more positive light. I thought about how grateful I was that science had made IVF possible. As I injected myself, I would consciously thank the injections and repeat positive affirmations.

During IVF, I grew very bloated as a result of the

progesterone I was taking, and I found that drinking plenty of water helped to ease this a little. Fresh mint tea was soothing, and gentle exercise such as yoga and walking also helped.

How did you respond when other people asked when you'd be starting a family?

The dreaded question that always felt like the elephant in the room. It's a deeply personal one and I was always taken aback when it came up, even when I knew it was being asked with the best intentions. Harry and I decided to come up with a standard reply so that we would never be left feeling upset or thinking about what we should be saying. We'd simply say, 'We're practising.' This was usually enough to give the message that perhaps things weren't so easy for us, and therefore it let the conversation move on to something else.

How did you remain hopeful in your pregnancy, following a miscarriage?

I still think of our miscarriage with deep sadness, and wonder about all that might have been. I've always felt so sorry that our little one didn't make it and ask myself whether it was something I did wrong or if it was my body that failed. Even though time's a healer, I'll never forget our loss.

I feel the experience of a miscarriage has made it more

difficult for me to relax during both of my pregnancies, but I always try to think positively and hold on to the hope that everything will be OK. I suppose once you've miscarried, you no longer have that innocent joy about pregnancy and you become more fearful of something going wrong.

Taking my pregnancy one day at a time and only looking as far ahead as the next milestone helped me to stay focused, although I don't think I relaxed fully until Lola was delivered safely into the world.

I've learned that the worries you have as a parent start right from the moment you find out you're pregnant – and never stop!

What's the greatest lesson your experience has taught you?

That there's always a lesson to be learned! Personally, the most important thing I've learned has been how to let go. Being in control has always been my way of coping with life, especially with my anxiety. Ironically, letting go has helped me to overcome some of my greatest fears.

I've also learned to live in the moment, not only when I was going through IVF treatment but also now that I'm a mum. When I'm with Lola I'm always in the present, thinking about what her needs are at that time. It's made me realize how much I used to exist in the past or in the future, and very rarely in the now! I believe that my whole journey towards meeting Lola happened for a reason, and feel it would be sad if I didn't try my best to learn from that.

Acknowledgements

A HUGE THANK YOU to Larry Finlay and everybody at Transworld Publishers who has been involved with *Dare to Dream*, particularly Becky Short, Helen Edwards, Alice Murphy-Pyle, Emma Burton, the design team, and my copy-editor, Becky Wright. I feel very lucky to have been given the opportunity to share my story and to have such a brilliant and committed team around me.

A special thank you to my editor Michelle Signore. From the moment we met I knew you understood me and you have continued to do so throughout the writing process. Thank you for your constant support and guidance – I'm so proud of what we have achieved together.

My wonderful agent, Steph Thwaites, who, right from the start, with no hesitation, made it possible for me to tell my story in the way I had always hoped. Thank you for your

Acknowledgements

dedication, sharing my vision and for always being at the end of the phone.

Thank you to Emily for helping me put my thoughts to paper in some sort of readable order! I will cherish the hours we shared talking (well, me talking and you listening). It has been the most therapeutic experience and a journey of discovery. It is thanks to you that I have been able to express myself and open up fully. I will be forever thankful to you. It has been a pleasure to write *Dare to Dream* with you.

Dr Ram Navaratnarajah of Babyinc. Ram, how can we begin to thank you. You are always willing to give up your own time to put your patients' needs first. Thank you for being the reassuring voice at the end of the phone and for going above and beyond. We will be eternally grateful to you.

To our fertility clinic, Herts & Essex – thank you for giving us a safe place. You made us feel confident at our most vulnerable time. Particularly, I would like to thank Soriah for all the time you gave us, the embryologists for your dedication and kindness and to the lovely Sarah for holding my hand.

Beth, thank you for helping me at a time when I felt so terrified and lonely. Within the space of a phone call you gave me so much courage and hope. It is thanks to you that I learned it is OK to put myself first sometimes.

To Lucy and the midwife-led team at Chelsea and Westminster Hospital, thank you for looking after us so beautifully. Especially to Ali – no words will ever truly describe the gratitude you feel to the person who delivers your baby safely into the world. I'm so happy to have found a friend for life in you.

Chunny, where to start? You are so much more than a best friend. I never knew how important it was to have someone like you in my life until I met you, now I don't know where I would be without you. Please let's never forget how to laugh together like we do and sit happily in silence together like we do! Thank you for being such a beautiful and loyal friend. You are the kindest soul I know.

To both our families, thank you for your unconditional love and support.

To Harry's family for being there for us both. Since day one I have felt like part of the family and you have all made me feel so loved. I'm very proud to call myself a Judd!

To Mum and Dad for your endless devotion and for teaching me how to keep going, no matter what life throws at me. I often think about your words 'make it happen' and 'dignity at all times'. Thank you for teaching me the strength of love.

Roops, you are the most loveable person I know. Anyone who is lucky enough to have you in their lives will be a happier person. You are a true inspiration to everyone and I'm so proud to call you my big brother.

Massey, you have continued to be the biggest comfort to me throughout my life. I don't know anyone else who cares so deeply about their family and who will drop everything to be there in times of need. We would all be very lost without you.

Guy, we will always be Darby and Joan! Thank you for always looking out for me and showing me that if you put your mind to something you can achieve anything. You are so kind to Lola, just as you have always been to me.

Acknowledgements

Harry, thank you for giving me the time to write *Dare to Dream* and for your endless support to make it possible. You are always there, quietly reassuring and encouraging me. Thank you for being my rational mind and for being so patient (I know I have been a little hormonal for a good few years now!). Without you this book would be nothing, as it was you who gave me the confidence to write my story. Thank you for making me feel complete and for being the best daddy and husband I could ever have wished for.

Lola, I can't believe someone so little has taught me so much. Since the day you were born you have been a ray of sunshine. Such a content, happy soul that brightens up everyone's day, but most of all mine. You are my everything and because of you my heart will always be filled with hope and love.

To the little one growing in my tummy, we are so excited to meet you. I know Lola will be such a devoted big sister to you. I will always believe *Dare to Dream* gave us you, thank you for helping me believe anything is possible.

And finally, to all the couples who have written to me over the months and often moved me to tears with their own stories. It is thanks to you that I was inspired to open up about our fertility struggles. You gave me the confidence to tell my story, so this is for you. I hope you find comfort and companionship in *Dare to Dream*. Please keep in touch and tell me all about your little miracles.

Never stop believing. Amazing things will happen.

AUTHOR BIOGRAPHY

Izzy Judd was born into a musical family in 1984. She studied the violin first at Chethams School of Music and then the Royal Academy of Music. She was a member of electric string quartet Escala, who took part in *Britain's Got Talent* in 2008 and went on to release a top-ten album with Simon Cowell's label SYCO. Izzy met Harry Judd on McFly's Wonderland tour in 2005 and they married in 2012. Izzy is now a full-time mum to their daughter Lola.

If you would like to carry on the conversation with Izzy, you can find her at MrsIzzyJudd (Facebook) and @mrs_izzyjudd (Instagram and Twitter)

PICTURE ACKNOWLEDGEMENTS

All photos courtesy of the author unless otherwise stated. Every effort has been made to contact the copyright holders. We apologize for any omissions in this respect and will be pleased to make the appropriate acknowledgements in any future edition.

Pages 1, 8, 10 and 42 © Sven Arnstein for *Hello!* magazine
Page 45 © Judith van Lent
Page 61 © Shaw Shots Photography (www.shawshots.com)
Pages 195 and 238 © David Spearing
Page 258 © Laura Beth Photography
    (www.laurabethphotography.co.uk)

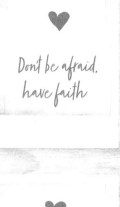

Don't be afraid,
have faith

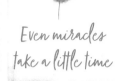

Even miracles
take a little time

Stay hopeful,
you never know
what tomorrow
may bring

BElieve in
YOUrself

Life can only be
understood backwards,
but it must be lived
forwards

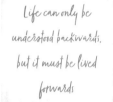

Trust the timing
of your life

Take time to do
what makes your
soul happy

And now I'll do
what's best for me

Life isn't about
waiting for the storm
to pass, it's about
learning to dance in
the rain

She took a
deep breath and
let it go

Tomorrow could be
the someday you've
been waiting for

Focus on
the good